OCD IN CHILDREN AND ADOLESCENTS

OCD in Children and Adolescents

The *"OCD Is Not the Boss of Me"* Manual

Katherine McKenney
Annie Simpson
S. Evelyn Stewart

THE GUILFORD PRESS
New York   London

Copyright © 2020 The Guilford Press
A Division of Guilford Publications, Inc.
370 Seventh Avenue, Suite 1200, New York, NY 10001
www.guilford.com

All rights reserved

Except as noted, no part of this book may be reproduced, translated, stored in a retrieval system, or transmitted, in any form or by any means, electronic, mechanical, photocopying, microfilming, recording, or otherwise, without written permission from the publisher.

Printed in the United States of America

This book is printed on acid-free paper.

Last digit is print number: 9   8   7   6   5   4   3   2   1

LIMITED DUPLICATION LICENSE

These materials are intended for use only by qualified mental health professionals.

The publisher grants to individual purchasers of this book nonassignable permission to reproduce all materials for which permission is specifically granted in a footnote. This license is limited to you, the individual purchaser, for personal use or use with children or youth and their parents. This license does not grant the right to reproduce these materials for resale, redistribution, electronic display, or any other purposes (including but not limited to books, pamphlets, articles, video- or audiotapes, blogs, file-sharing sites, Internet or intranet sites, and handouts or slides for lectures, workshops, or webinars, whether or not a fee is charged). Permission to reproduce these materials for these and any other purposes must be obtained in writing from the Permissions Department of Guilford Publications.

The authors have checked with sources believed to be reliable in their efforts to provide information that is complete and generally in accord with the standards of practice that are accepted at the time of publication. However, in view of the possibility of human error or changes in behavioral, mental health, or medical sciences, neither the authors, nor the editors and publisher, nor any other party who has been involved in the preparation or publication of this work warrants that the information contained herein is in every respect accurate or complete, and they are not responsible for any errors or omissions or the results obtained from the use of such information. Readers are encouraged to confirm the information contained in this book with other sources.

Library of Congress Cataloging-in-Publication data

Names: McKenney, Katherine, author. | Simpson, Annie, author. | Stewart, S. Evelyn, author.
Title: OCD in children and adolescents : the "OCD is not the boss of me" manual / Katherine McKenney, Annie Simpson, S. Evelyn Stewart.
Description: New York : The Guilford Press, 2020. | Includes bibliographical references and index. |
Identifiers: LCCN 2019043404 | ISBN 9781462542031 (paperback) | ISBN 9781462542048 (hardcover)
Subjects: LCSH: Obsessive–compulsive disorder in children—Treatment. | Obsessive–compulsive disorder in adolescence—Treatment. | Cognitive therapy.
Classification: LCC RJ506.O25 M382 2019 | DDC 616.85/22700835—dc23
LC record available at *https://lccn.loc.gov/2019043404*

Illustrations by Matthew Ferguson

About the Authors

Katherine McKenney, PhD, is a staff psychologist with the Provincial OCD Clinic and Research Program at BC Children's Hospital (BCCH) in Vancouver, British Columbia, Canada, as well as Adjunct Professor in the Department of Psychology at the University of British Columbia and a director at Cornerstone Child and Family Psychology Clinic. At BCCH, Dr. McKenney provides assessment and group treatment to youth with obsessive–compulsive disorder (OCD) and their families. She also consults and trains clinicians around the province, is actively involved in research and program development, and has coauthored numerous peer-reviewed publications. Dr. McKenney has developed several group therapy manuals for the treatment of OCD and maintains a busy private practice.

Annie Simpson, PhD, is a director at Cornerstone Child and Family Psychology Clinic and a clinical associate in the Department of Psychology at Simon Fraser University in Burnaby, British Columbia. She previously worked as a staff psychologist with the Provincial OCD Clinic and Research Program at BCCH. Dr. Simpson was actively involved in research and program development in her role at BCCH and coauthored numerous publications. She has worked as a consultant for Anxiety Canada, providing lectures and workshops and developing self-help materials for children and adolescents.

S. Evelyn Stewart, MD, is Full Professor in the Department of Psychiatry at the University of British Columbia and Founding Director of the Provincial OCD Clinic and Research Program at BCCH, the first integrated clinic and research program for pediatric OCD in Canada. Dr. Stewart spent her early career as a psychiatrist within the pediatric and adult OCD clinic teams at Massachusetts General Hospital, as Research Director of the OCD Institute at McLean Hospital, and as Assistant Professor at Harvard Medical School. She has authored over 100 original papers, reviews, and book chapters on family, genetic, neuroimaging, and treatment aspects of OCD and related illnesses throughout the life-span.

Preface

In 2011, an interdisciplinary group of clinicians came together at British Columbia Children's Hospital to create the first combined pediatric obsessive–compulsive disorder (OCD) clinic and research program in Canada. Consisting of psychology, child and adolescent psychiatry, and social work clinicians and neuroscience researchers, the team brought together expertise from complementary realms.

Since that time, we have had the privilege of providing comprehensive assessment and treatment to hundreds of OCD-affected children and youth and their families. We have typically provided cognitive-behavioral therapy (CBT) in concurrent group settings, using either weekly or daily intensive formats. This book is the product of an iterative process that has taken place since the founding of our program. Changes in our treatment approach have been guided by feedback from data-driven research, but, more important, from the children, youth, and families undertaking their treatment journey with us.

Notably, parent involvement is a mandatory, central part of the process. As clinicians, we partner with both parents and their OCD-affected children as they engage in exposure and response prevention (ERP) skill building. For the children and youth, this involves exposure to core OCD fears with refusal to subsequently engage in what have typically been longstanding, ingrained rituals. For the parents, this involves exposure to their child's OCD-related distress as they practice ERP, followed by a host of novel responses, which may include refusal to accommodate or empathic support to join with the child in their fight against "the OCD bully."

Throughout the years, we have repeatedly been told stories of families unable to access OCD-focused ERP treatment, which is the best empirically proven first-line approach for pediatric OCD. We have also noted the many families who unknowingly invest significant resources (via time and finances) toward non-evidence-based care for their children, including relaxation training and insight-oriented and attachment-based treatments for OCD. Given that early access to appropriate treatment predicts long-term outcome, this has been particularly discouraging to hear. It also spawned the idea for this book.

Our program was founded with a mandate to address OCD in children and youth across the province of British Columbia in Canada, a landmass greater in area than England and France combined, and twice the size of California. We have hosted OCD CBT training events run by the International OCD Foundation and subsequently by our own team members, and regularly invite community mental health team members to observe and participate with our groups. In discussions with community-based clinicians near and far, it became clear that they often felt intimidated and ill-equipped to work with OCD-affected children and youth.

OCD affects approximately 1–3% of children and adolescents, and does not tend to self-resolve over time. However, it is clear that early intervention for all new-onset cases in tertiary care subspecialty settings is neither feasible nor desirable. As such, an "army" of ERP-trained therapists is required within communities to mitigate the negative effects of this illness.

Our goal for this book was to create a readily accessible resource that would empower clinicians to embrace nonpharmacological CBT treatment of pediatric OCD. We drew on collective experience of more than 40 years to write a clinician-friendly book that will guide therapists through a standard treatment protocol and also provide clinical pearls of wisdom and share lessons learned from our past successes (and errors!). An extensive variety of exposure ideas is provided for different OCD symptom presentations and developmental stages of affected children and youth.

This book comprises a "preparing for treatment" section (Part I), followed by a 10-module manual (Part II) that allows you to flexibly approach evidence-based treatment with children, youth, and their parents in an engaging and family-centered manner. Module content is based on sessions provided during our weekly and intensive groups. Reproducible parent and child/youth handouts and worksheets accompany each module. (See the box at the end of the table of contents.) Through integrated research within our clinical program, we have been able to identify clinically and statistically significant changes following treatment. These include improvements reported from child, parent, and clinician perspectives across a multitude of domains, including OCD severity, personal and family impacts, accommodation (Selles et al., 2018a), and OCD-related coercive/disruptive behaviors (Schuberth, Selles, & Stewart, 2018). Thus, in stark contrast to the treatment landscape for many childhood mental illnesses, an effective, efficient, and structured treatment approach is available for OCD that can transform the lives of affected children and youth and their families.

Working with families in helping them to overcome OCD has been a personal and professional source of great joy in each of our lives. We hope the following pages will demystify OCD-focused CBT treatment, allowing you to discover how fun and rewarding this therapeutic work truly is.

Intended Audience

This book is written for mental health clinicians working with OCD-affected children and adolescents, and specifically for those in search of a detailed and structured approach to treating this disorder. Given the heterogeneity of OCD symptom types, many clinical case examples (all fictional/composite based on the many different children, youth, and families we have treated over the years) and sample scripts and dialogues have intentionally been provided to increase clinician self-confidence in managing the variety of OCD-related issues emerging in treatment.

It is expected that the readership of this book will have both a general background in child mental health treatment and prior knowledge of CBT principles and their application. From those currently struggling with their first OCD management case to those who have previously treated dozens or more of OCD-affected children and youth, we hope this book will provide guidance and novel ideas as you navigate the tricky yet rewarding treatment of OCD. Based on our own experience, and regardless of the reader's formal expertise, we also recommend regular peer consultation with other OCD clinicians to support your work and practice.

How to Use This Book

This book has two parts. Part I provides clinicians with an overview of OCD and its evidence-based treatment as foundational knowledge and background to build upon with the treatment skills described in the second part of the book. We strongly encourage clinicians who are new to the treatment of OCD to read Part I before proceeding with the treatment modules.

Part II of the book consists of 10 treatment modules, covering a variety of aspects and components involved in the treatment of OCD, with primary emphasis on ERP techniques. Each module focuses on a specific OCD treatment-related topic, with suggestions on how it should be addressed, descriptions of related therapeutic techniques, and selected anecdotal "tips and tricks" collected by us over our careers. The modules are designed to be used flexibly. If you happen to be newly starting treatment with a family, you may wish to proceed through the modules in order. In contrast, you may focus on specific modules for families who have been in treatment for some time, or for whom only some aspects of the treatment protocol are relevant. Module worksheets and handouts for parents and children/youth are included for use in session or to assign as homework. Our hope is that this book will provide clinicians with the practical advice and specific ERP examples for which they have been searching.

A Note on Language

In this book, when referring to a child or youth, we use "they/them/their" as a singular pronoun. We have made this choice to be inclusive of those who do not identify with masculine/feminine pronouns.

Acknowledgments

Katherine McKenney: This book would not exist without the help and inspiration of the families with whom I work. I am in awe of the strength and resilience of parents and youth with OCD, and I consider it a privilege to help them reclaim their lives from this disorder. I want to express my appreciation to The Guilford Press, particularly Kitty Moore and Barbara Watkins, for their guidance, feedback, and cheerleading of this project. Thank you to Dr. Daniel Lafleur for his thoughtful feedback on an earlier version of the manuscript. I am grateful for the creativity and wisdom of my coauthors, Annie and Evelyn. I can't imagine writing this book with anyone else. I am so proud of what we've created together, and I hope it will accomplish our goal: to ensure more children with OCD can access effective and evidence-based treatment. Finally, I would like to thank my parents for helping me believe I can do anything I set my mind to; my husband, Matt, for giving me the time, support, and encouragement to write this book; and my daughters, Emma and Sophie, for always helping me find the fun in life.

Annie Simpson: Treating OCD has been one of the most rewarding parts of my career so far. I'm so grateful to the families with children with OCD who have allowed me to be a part of their journey and the tremendous amount of knowledge I have gained. This book is a direct result of those experiences. Thank you to the team at The Guilford Press for their ongoing support. Thank you to Evelyn for providing me with this wonderful opportunity to share our knowledge with others so more kids can live without the burden of OCD. And Katherine—there is no one else I would want to (or could) write a book with! I'm truly grateful for our 20-plus-year friendship! Last, I want to thank my children, Lev and Tali. It's not easy having a "brave" doctor for a mom! I love you guys so much.

S. Evelyn Stewart: Great gratitude is owed to the many individuals contributing to this book's creation. To Kitty Moore and The Guilford Press for your trust and patience and to Dr. John Walkup for connecting us. To early mentors who introduced me to the rewards, privileges, and challenges of working in the fight against OCD: Drs. Peter Boyle, Michael Jenike, and Scott Rauch. To McLean OCD Institute and International OCD Foundation colleagues. To the multitalented and dedicated BCCH Provincial OCD Program team, and to those administrative leaders, donors, and families who have supported its foundation and growth. To OCDbc and Anxiety Canada. On a personal note, I thank my parents for instilling in me a belief that nothing is impossible and the crucial goal to do my best no matter what; my husband, Michael DeMarni, for being "my person" on our life adventures; and our five children—Chiara, Emmi, Lorenzo, Gabrielle, and Luca—who continue to amaze and teach me about the resiliency of youth, and the importance of treating everyone with a view of their amazing and unique strengths and challenges.

Witnessing the burden endured and the resiliency displayed by OCD-affected children, youth, adults, and their families has been a driving and inspiring force for me throughout my career. Despite advances in other aspects of OCD research, notable gains have been limited in recent decades with respect to improving access to treatment and the lived experience of those with OCD. Effectiveness of ERP techniques in first-line treatment of OCD is old news in 2020. Yet, overwhelming barriers to ERP access persist, driven by health care and insurance system factors, in addition to undertrained community providers. It is my sincere hope that this book helps to decrease access barriers by helping to demystify OCD treatment.

Contents

PART I. Preparing to Initiate Exposure and Response Prevention   1

CHAPTER 1. An Overview of Pediatric Obsessive–Compulsive Disorder and Its Treatment   3

CHAPTER 2. ERP Preparation and Delivery   13

CHAPTER 3. Fine-Tuning ERP Delivery   19

CHAPTER 4. Complementary Approaches to ERP   27

PART II. Providing Treatment: 10 Nuts-and-Bolts Modules   39

MODULE 1. Treatment Preparation with the Child or Youth and Their Parents   41

MODULE 2. Explaining ERPs, Building an OCD Ladder, and Implementing Rewards   70

MODULE 3. Foundational Treatment Tools: Breaking Free of OCD's Traps, Bossing Back OCD, and Identifying Family Accommodation   99

MODULE 4. Breaking OCD's Rules: The Four *S*'s, Exposure Games, and Limiting Family Accommodation and Reassurance Seeking   118

MODULE 5. Tools to Help with OCD "Bad Thoughts": Imaginal Exposures and Dealing with OCD-Related Rage   142

MODULE 6.	Tools to Help with ERPs: Coping Cards, Floating On By, Coping with Doubt Scripts, and Reducing Stigma	160
MODULE 7.	Troubleshooting ERPs: Suboptimal Response, Therapist Pitfalls, and Barriers to Treatment Success	177
MODULE 8.	Self- and Family Care: Boosting Self-Esteem, Attending to Personal Needs, and Managing OCD in Schools	195
MODULE 9.	Preparing for the Future: Relapse Prevention and Consolidating Gains	211
MODULE 10.	Graduation: Celebration and Maintenance of Gains	227
	References	243
	Index	249

Purchasers of this book can download and print additional copies of the handouts and worksheets, in color, at *www.guilford.com/mckenney-forms* for personal use or use with children or youth and their parents (see copyright page for details).

PART I
Preparing to Initiate Exposure and Response Prevention

CHAPTER 1

An Overview of Pediatric Obsessive–Compulsive Disorder and Its Treatment

What Is Pediatric OCD?

Obsessive–compulsive disorder (OCD) is one of the most debilitating mental disorders of our era, with half of cases striking in childhood (Westwell-Roper & Stewart, 2019). Delays in proper diagnosis and treatment of this disorder often extend over months or years. And, when left untreated, OCD tends to worsen due to negative reinforcement, leaving in its wake disrupted development, impeded academic and career achievement, and relationship difficulties (Fineberg et al., 2019). Yet, OCD has been proven responsive to skillfully conducted evidence-based treatment (Dougherty et al., 2018). Thus, despite being a severe illness, OCD is highly rewarding to treat given its potential for dramatic improvement within a limited time frame.

OCD Is Common

In the National Comorbidity Survey Replication, over one quarter (28.2%) of respondents reported having had an obsession or compulsion in their lifetime (Ruscio, Stein, Chiu, & Kessler, 2010). A smaller proportion of individuals in the population (1–3%) have full-blown OCD, involving functional impairment, significant distress, or notable time spent consumed by symptoms.

OCD Symptoms Are Diverse (and Often Misdiagnosed)

OCD is possibly one of the most misunderstood and underestimated disorders by the general public, given the familiarity of symptoms in their mild form (e.g., checking that a door is locked, washing hands in a particular pattern). The expression "I'm SO OCD" is both common and misleading, falsely suggesting that OCD is a positive personal characteristic rather than a debilitating, time-consuming, and biologically driven disease. In contrast to many other mental illnesses, OCD has symptom types that are very numerous and diverse. The Children's Yale–Brown Obsessive Compulsive Scale (CY-BOCS) checklist provides a list of over 70 symptom types across 13 categories of obsession and compulsion (Scahill et al., 1997).

In addition to the frequent co-occurrence of symptoms at a specific point of time, OCD symptoms in any given individual often change over the course of illness. A notable area of research interest has examined co-occurrence of OCD symptom types, known as symptom dimensions, within clinical and population samples (Stewart et al., 2008; Bloch, Landeros-Weisenberger, Rosario, Pittenger, & Leckman, 2008; Alvarenga et al., 2015).

Primary symptom factors or dimensions identified in pediatric OCD are as follows:

- *"Classic" OCD symptom dimension:* Contamination and somatic obsessions and cleaning compulsions.
- *"Intrusive thoughts" OCD symptom dimension:* Aggressive, sexual, and religious obsessions.
- *"Just-right" OCD symptom dimension:* Symmetry obsessions, ordering, repeating, counting, checking, and hoarding.

Symptom dimensions identified in adult OCD are very similar to those in pediatric OCD, with the exception that somatic and checking symptoms both move to the "bad thoughts" dimension, from the "classic" and "just-right" dimensions, respectively (Bloch et al., 2008). Moreover, "just right" and hoarding symptoms occupy separate factors in some related analyses.

While it was previously believed that limited insight is the "norm" in pediatric OCD, a recent meta-analysis by our team and international colleagues found that almost 90% had insight ranging between fair and excellent (Selles et al., 2018b).

OCD Comorbidity

Co-occurrence of additional mental illnesses are the rule rather than the exception in pediatric OCD. More than half of cases in epidemiological samples have at least one such comorbid illness (Flament et al., 1988). Comorbidities associated with earlier OCD onset include anxiety disorders, attention-deficit/hyperactivity disorder (ADHD), and tic disorders, whereas those associated with older OCD onset include mood and psychotic disorders (Geller et al., 2000).

OCD "Look-Alikes"

When a child or youth presents with repetitive behaviors or recurrent distressing thoughts and a presumed OCD diagnosis, it is important to ensure that these do not solely represent other diagnoses before proceeding with OCD-focused treatment approaches. Other childhood-onset illnesses with repetitive behaviors presenting as core symptoms include tic and autism spectrum disorders. Impairing adolescent-onset repetitive behaviors often present in the context of eating or obsessive–compulsive-related disorders (OCRDs; Coelho et al., 2019; Westwell-Roper & Stewart, 2019).

Alternative diagnoses to consider when assessing youth who present with distressing thoughts, related impairment, and presumed OCD include anxiety and psychotic disorders. However, due to OCD-driven secrecy, magical thinking, and the "oddness" of certain rituals, misdiagnoses between OCD and first-episode psychosis are too common, especially among adolescent males.

Specific, Complex, and Dramatic Acute-Onset Presentations

An OCD-related topic of controversy and recurring media attention over the past decade and a half relates to pediatric autoimmune neuropsychiatric disorders associated with streptococcal infections (PANDAS) and pediatric acute-onset neuropsychiatric syndrome (PANS) (Murphy, Gerardi, & Leckman, 2014). These are implicated when rapid and dramatic emergence of OCD (or tics or food restriction) occurs with a cluster of other newly occurring "non-OCD" symptoms. They have been noted to occur in 2–5% of pediatric OCD cases (Jaspers-Fayer et al., 2017). Parents are particularly vulnerable, as related family impairment is significantly higher than that in non-PANDAS/PANS cases of OCD (Jaspers-Fayer et al., 2017). Unfortunately, families seeking help often receive contradictory and alarming advice from professionals, paraprofessionals, and Internet sources with respect to best assessment and management of these presentations.

Diagnostic criteria for PANDAS and PANS are as follows:

PANDAS

- OCD and/or tic disorder
- Pediatric onset—between 3 years and puberty
- Abrupt onset or dramatic symptom exacerbation with a sawtooth course
- Association with a confirmed streptococcal infection
- Association with other neuropsychiatric symptoms (e.g., choreiform movements)

PANS

- Abrupt, dramatic onset of OCD symptoms or severe food intake restriction
- Concurrent, sudden onset of at least two of the following symptoms:
  - Anxiety
  - Emotional lability/depression
  - Irritability
  - Aggression and/or oppositional behaviors
  - Behavioral (developmental) regression
  - Deterioration in school performance

- Sensorimotor abnormalities
- Somatic signs and symptoms
* Symptoms not better explained by a known neurological or medical condition

OCD Often Begins in Childhood

OCD tends to emerge earlier in boys than girls. In males, onset peaks occur between 8 and 10 years, 18 and 22 years, and during the late 20s (Ruscio et al., 2010). In females, many cases onset between 20 and 30 years of age. These may coincide with periods of hormonal shifts that impact brain development and with times of major life transitions. While some cases of new OCD onset are reported in the elderly, this is uncommon.

It has been suggested that childhood-onset OCD may represent a distinct subtype of the disorder (Chabane et al., 2005). This group has higher rates of comorbid tics and ADHD. In addition, the role of genetics appears to be stronger in the childhood-onset form, being responsible for approximately 45–65% of attributable risk, compared to 27–47% in adults (van Grootheest, Cath, Beekman, & Boomsma, 2005). However, despite international efforts, no specific OCD risk genes have been confirmed (Dougherty et al., 2018).

OCD Symptoms and Avoidance Are Debilitating

It is estimated that an average of 3 years of wages are lost over the lifetime of those with OCD due to this illness (Hollander & Wong, 1995), and that those experiencing OCD spend an average of 10 hours a day engaging in OCD symptoms (Ruscio et al., 2010). Quality of life (Coluccia, Ferretti, Fagiolini, & Pozza, 2017), sleep (Jaspers-Fayer et al., 2018), athletic (Cromer, Kaier, Davis, Stunk, & Stewart, 2017) and academic function (Negreiros, Belschner, Selles, Lin, & Stewart, 2018; Perez-Vigil et al., 2018) are also negatively impacted by OCD. Fortunately, prompt intervention and treatment in childhood and adolescence can positively impact the long-term trajectory of OCD and enhance the well-being of children, youth, and families impacted by OCD (Fineberg et al., 2019).

OCD Prognosis

While adult OCD has historically been considered a chronic diagnosis, facts suggest that the childhood-onset form of this illness (especially when associated with tics) has a better long-term prognosis (Bloch et al., 2009). Based on independent study samples, less than one-half of children (41%) have ongoing OCD at long-term follow-up and approximately 20% have only nonimpairing OCD symptoms (Micali et al., 2010; Stewart et al., 2004). Of interest, it is not severity of OCD symptoms, but rather the duration of illness prior to assessment that predicts persistence (Stewart et al., 2004; Melin, Skarphedinsson, Skärsäter, Haugland, & Ivarsson, 2018). Thus, it is important to emphasize to parents (and to clinicians!) that early recognition and intervention are important to optimize their child's outcome. This has been emphasized in a 2019 international expert consensus statement (Fineberg et al., 2019). In addition, it is crucial to remember that OCD can be well managed despite occasional, intermittent recurrence of symptoms.

Family Accommodation and Impacts

While all childhood illnesses have an impact on families, pediatric OCD is especially impairing. OCD symptoms frequently involve and demand participation or accommodation by family members and others living in the home. In fact, over 90% of OCD-affected families report accommodating to either prevent or relieve their relative's OCD-triggered distress (Stewart et al., 2008).

Family accommodation includes compulsion facilitation (e.g., listening to "confessions"), reassurance giving, and enabling avoidance of triggers (e.g., abstaining from saying certain words; Peris et al., 2008). Although well intentioned, family accommodation inadvertently worsens OCD symptoms and is associated with increased disease severity, higher functional impairment, and poor treatment response (Storch et al., 2007a). While family accommodation behaviors are often performed without awareness of their negative impacts, even engaged and committed parents frequently struggle to resist accommodating in acute situations due to the difficulty of tolerating their child's acute OCD-related distress.

Regardless of family accommodation, general impacts of OCD on family life are extensive (Stewart et al., 2017). The burden on caregivers of adults with OCD is comparable to that of caregivers of those with schizophrenia (Thomas, Suresh Kujmar, Verma, Sinha, & Andrade, 2004). Moreover, burden and negative impacts on quality of life have been noted for parents of OCD-affected youth (Wu et al., 2018).

The family activities most commonly impacted by childhood OCD include morning and bedtime routines and mealtimes. Compared to families of those with clinical depression, families of OCD-affected individuals experience greater illness burden and more impaired functioning, partially due to the increased expressed anger when illness-related demands are not accommodated. Nearly one-half of mothers and a third of fathers report daily impacts on their jobs due to their child's OCD symptoms. Moreover, over half of parents reported that they often or always feel anxious, frustrated, and saddened by their child's OCD.

Treatment of Pediatric OCD

OCD Improves with Treatment

OCD-affected families and their clinicians are currently in a much better position than their predecessors 30–40 years ago. This is thanks to a plethora of pediatric and adult OCD studies demonstrating the efficacy of both cognitive-behavioral therapy (CBT) and serotonin reuptake inhibitor medications, including selective serotonin reuptake inhibitors (SSRIs) and clomipramine (Bloch & Storch, 2015).

The Pediatric OCD Treatment Study (POTS) is the landmark study comparing medication, CBT, and combined approaches with placebo in pediatric OCD management (Pediatric OCD Treatment Study Team, 2004). The CBT treatment regimen involved 14 1-hour therapy sessions over 12 weeks, including psychoeducation, cognitive training, OCD symptom mapping, and exposure and response prevention (ERP). The latter component represents a core element in the psychosocial treatment of OCD and involves having the child or youth gradually and systematically confront their feared OCD triggers *without* engaging in the rituals that previously were employed to reduce anxiety or other distressing emotions that the stimulus caused. With repeated exposure, the child habituates to the stimulus and the urge to engage in the ritual dissipates. Reported remission rates and number needed to treat (NNT) data (number of individuals required to receive treatment to expect OCD remission in one individual) were as follows: sertraline (21%, NNT = 5.6); CBT (39%, NNT = 2.8); and combined sertraline + CBT (54%, NNT = 2.0), versus placebo (4%). While some debate remains with respect to the relative efficacy of combined treatment (CBT and medication) versus either CBT alone or medication alone in pediatric OCD, a consistently replicated fact is that CBT (with and without medication) is statistically and clinically superior to placebo (Westwell-Roper & Stewart, 2019).

OCD Is Rewarding to Treat

OCD is a rewarding condition to treat, with frequent success stories and happy, very grateful families. However, the complexity, changing nature, and subtlety of OCD symptoms can provide challenges to provision of high-quality CBT. There is no "one-size-fits-all" approach, and clinician skill and creativity are assets when developing ERP activities. This fact was demonstrated by the results of the POTS trial, which reflected the importance of individual CBT skills as an influence on outcomes. Specifically, observed treatment effect sizes differed notably across sites for CBT (0.5–1.6, ranging widely from medium to very large effect), whereas this was not found for sertraline (0.5–0.8, medium effect across all sites).

While OCD recognition and diagnosis have improved, and while ERP is clearly proven for use across the life-span, sadly only a minority of affected individuals access this treatment. One of the largest barriers to access has been created by limited availability of CBT providers trained in ERP for OCD. This book has been written in an effort to increase the confidence and willingness of CBT-trained clinicians to embark on the rewarding journey of becoming an OCD therapist!

How ERP works

ERP has long persisted as the most effective therapeutic approach in the treatment of OCD. It appears that there is more than one mechanism by which improvements occur, including both habituation and inhibitory learning (Hezel & Simpson, 2019).

The treatment program presented in this book, and in leading pediatric and adult OCD CBT books historically, is largely based upon the premise that a process called habituation is at play. This idea, as proposed by Foa's emotional processing theory, states that exposures work when the fear or distress evoked by a stimulus (i.e., "fear response") decreases as that stimulus is repeatedly presented (Foa & Kozak, 1986). This may occur both within and between practice sessions. Guided by this theory, traditional ERP paradigms involve systematic exposure to progressive, increasingly challenging stimuli after each has been "mastered" (i.e., has lost the ability to trigger a fear response).

Recent years have added clarity regarding ERP mechanisms in OCD. Driven by the formidable work of Michelle Craske (e.g., Craske, Treanor, Conway, Zbozinek, & Vervliet, 2014), inhibitory learning (IL) theory suggests that the initial fear response is not extinguished, forgotten, or unlearned. The fear response continues to be evoked. However, during exposure, a tolerance of the subsequent experience of discomfort or distress occurs, and this new response inhibits or overrides the old response.

So, how does this impact specific aspects of ERP treatment for OCD or anxiety? Discussion of habituation versus inhibitory learning mechanisms is more than only theoretical. As noted, a spirit of creativity, curiosity, willingness to learn, and persistence through iterative trial and error are tools used by the best OCD ERP treatment providers. It is likely that both extinction and inhibitory learning are in play during ERP.

Some children do not report progressive decreases in anxiety with ERP. From an IL perspective, this does not necessarily mean the therapy is not working, given that new learning is still taking place. What the children or youth may be developing in these cases are new expectations of how bad the feared stimulus will be and how capable they are at tolerating the related distress. For these children or youth, measuring numerical ratings of distress (subjective units of distress [SUDs]; see Module 1) is not particularly useful, nor is working on a graduated fear ladder. Instead, varying the intensity of exposures and the settings in which they occur may promote more generalization of the learning process.

Of note, most of the modules in this book are based on emotional processing theory and habituation. Module adaptations based on IL theory as described previously may be used as deemed appropriate, especially for cases in which habituation does not appear to be occurring.

Generalizing ERP Successes

An important aspect in the treatment of pediatric OCD is the generalization of gains made in the treatment session to the regular life environment. While it is wonderful when a child or youth is able to touch door handles in the office and to resist handwashing for the first time, that does little to impact day-to-day functioning if similar gains do not extend to their home, school, or community. For this reason, ERP exercises are often most effective when conducted outside of the clinician's office. This can include completing ERPs while riding public transit with a child or youth, visiting public restrooms together, visiting places of worship, or having them touch contaminated objects in their home.

Every clinician may not have the capacity to complete ERPs outside the office, either due to geographical limitations or occupational restrictions. One way to overcome this barrier is to have youth and families bring in obsessional triggers from home (e.g., contaminated clothing, a Bible, items that need to be organized in a specific way) and to use them in session. Similarly, between-session homework can be developed so that children or youth have opportunities to complete ERPs in a variety of triggering settings. For example, if they have difficulties touching bathroom taps, then over the course of treatment they should be completing ERPs that include touching taps at home, at friends' houses, at the mall, and at school (depending on identified related obsessional triggers). Families should be asked to plan on dedicating at least a half hour of homework each day to focusing on exposures and response prevention. For some families, this may necessitate helping parents to carve out time by eliminating selected extracurricular activities during the active treatment period.

When to Consider Alternatives or to Temporarily Delay ERPs

A majority of children and youth respond positively to ERPs and experience a decrease in OCD symptoms through processes that likely include habituation or inhibitory learning, as described previously. While it is impossible to predict outcomes for individual children or youth, certain identifiable factors influence the likelihood of CBT success.

A recent systematic review found that comorbid tics and a family history of OCD moderate CBT treatment response in pediatric OCD (Turner, O'Gorman, Nair, & O'Kearney, 2018). Compared to placebo response rates, children with tics were more likely to respond to CBT alone but not to an SSRI (sertraline) alone. However, for initial CBT nonresponders, the presence of tics favored addition of sertraline over continued CBT alone.

Those with a family history of OCD were more likely to respond to CBT combined with an SSRI (sertraline), but not to CBT alone. Other factors associated with poorer CBT response included older age, OCD severity, comorbidity, and increased family accommodation. The following may be a helpful guideline for individual cases. Appropriate treatment includes reduction of avoidance and family accommodation, and:

- Mild OCD → CBT alone
- Moderate to severe OCD:
    - Family history of OCD → CBT + SSRI
    - Comorbid tics → CBT alone → if non-response, add SSRI
    - No OCD family history or comorbid tics → CBT ± SSRI

For a small percentage of OCD-affected children and youth, significant and risky maladaptive behaviors may emerge or worsen in the context of ERP treatment. Those with uncontrolled patterns of behavior including self-injurious acts, violence, suicide attempts, or substance use may turn to these as a means of coping with ERP-triggered distress. Blindly continuing to encourage ERPs for these individuals without adequate emotion regulation skills and adaptive coping is unwise, as treatment will likely further exacerbate unsafe behaviors. Continuing will effectively distract from OCD treatment targets and enable avoidance. In such circumstances, it is often best to suspend ERP and shift the focus to adaptive coping and emotion regulation skill development. This may involve utilizing a dialectical behavior therapy (DBT)-informed approach or referring the individual to a DBT specialty program, with a long-term plan to return and engage in OCD-focused ERP. However, it is important to send a message to the family that the long-term goal is for the child or youth to eventually engage in ERP, once they have developed the skills necessary for this challenge.

Being Aware of Inappropriate (and Potentially Therapist-Related) ERP Delays

Despite the potential problems noted above, it is important to not "enable" ongoing delays leading up to ERP initiation. In our experience, it is far more common for therapists to spend inappropriately long periods of time prior to initiating ERPs while conducting background assessment and supportive therapy than it is for them to begin ERPs inappropriately early. Baseline factors such as limited insight and the presence of coercive behaviors have historically been identified as reasons to be skeptical about potential ERP success. However, these notions have been challenged by findings that both coercive behavior and insight level tend to improve with ERP in childhood OCD (Selles et al., 2018a). In fact, improvement in coercive/disruptive behavior predicts OCD severity and individual and family functioning improvement (Schuberth, Selles, & Stewart, 2018). Moreover, the presence of poor insight does not appear to predict CBT nonresponse, although the absence of insight does predict CBT dropout (Selles et al., 2019).

Delays to initiating ERPs may also reflect therapist hesitancy and unwitting avoidance of the inevitable related distress witnessed in the youth, and at times experienced by the therapist. While it is natural for therapists (who have committed themselves to a career of helping others, after all!) to hesitate prior to ERP initiation, it is important to not overvalue the meaning or true danger of OCD-related distress. Such delays may signal to the child or youth (and parents) that they are not strong enough to face up to the OCD bully.

Overview of the "OCD Is Not the Boss of Me" Treatment Program

Part II of this book consists of 10 treatment modules covering a variety of topics in the treatment of OCD, with primary emphasis on ERP techniques. The module topics are as follows:

- Module 1: Treatment Preparation with the Child or Youth and Their Parents
- Module 2: Explaining ERPs, Building an OCD Ladder, and Implementing Rewards
- Module 3: Foundational Treatment Tools
- Module 4: Breaking OCD's Rules
- Module 5: Tools to Help with OCD "Bad Thoughts"
- Module 6: Tools to Help with ERPs
- Module 7: Troubleshooting ERPs
- Module 8: Self- and Family Care
- Module 9: Preparing for the Future
- Module 10: Graduation

These modules are designed for flexible use with children, youth, and families to allow for an individualized treatment approach. When initiating treatment, it may be most helpful to proceed in chronological order through the modules, recognizing that some modules may be covered in a single session whereas others may require multiple sessions, as influenced by symptom presentation, treatment engagement, and individual specifics. For treatment that is already under way with OCD-affected children or youth, it may be prudent to skip ahead to modules that are most relevant at a given time.

Modules may be used selectively. Pacing of treatment is based upon clinical judgment, child and youth motivation and engagement, parent buy-in, session frequency and intensity, and between-session progress. Modules are intended to inspire confidence when treating pediatric OCD via ERP. We have intentionally included many case examples within modules to provide descriptions of how tools can be used selectively based upon clinical judgment.

Each module focuses on a specific OCD treatment-related topic, with suggestions on how to present this information to families, and selected pearls of wisdom accumulated by the authors. Reproducible parent and child/youth worksheets and handouts accompany each module. (See the box at the end of the table of contents.) Anecdotally, treatment approaches that are primarily behavioral in nature tend to result in the best outcomes for children and youth with OCD. Although some cognitive strategies have been included in the modules (e.g., *bossing back the OCD bully; coping cards*), the emphasis of "OCD Is Not the Boss of Me" is focused on ERP activities. The use of cognitive approaches that focus on recognizing faulty cognitions can leave the patient stuck in arguments about the "What ifs" (e.g., "What if I get HIV?" "What if I go to hell?" "What if I left the stove on?"). This is particularly the case if the clinician's emphasis is on attempting to challenge or change the content of the obsessions (e.g., "There's a very low chance that I left the stove on"). OCD is associated with poor tolerance of uncertainty (Hezel, Stewart, McNally, & Riemann, 2019). No outcome can be guaranteed with 100% certainty, so discussions around the likelihood of an outcome can leave children and youth focused on the 0.00001% chance of something bad happening to them. In addition, studies consistently demonstrate that exposure is the key element in overcoming anxiety, including OCD.

CHAPTER 2

ERP Preparation and Delivery

Before beginning ERPs with a child or youth, clinicians need to gather some specific information about the OCD presentation and related involvement of family members. Jumping into treatment without this knowledge can result in slower treatment progress, ineffective ERPs, and subsequently decreased child or youth engagement.

Preparing to engage on the ERP treatment path with children, youth, and their parents is important. This will provide a realistic understanding of what to expect, and what will be expected of them. Families with past treatment experience in other therapeutic modalities may understandably expect that the majority of session time will be dedicated to the reporting and processing of emotions raised by OCD and related events since the previous session. However, ERP sessions should have less emphasis on self-reflection and greater emphasis on skill building, including in-session practicing. A sample 50-minute session outline is as follows:

- Check-in: 5 minutes.
- Review of homework: 5 minutes.
- Teaching the OCD strategy: 10 minutes.
- ERP practice: 20 minutes.
- Homework assignment/reward: 10 minutes.

Below you will find a summary of specific questions to help develop an effective treatment plan. For children or youth with many OCD symptoms, clinicians have the option to focus on one symptom area initially, gathering information about that before proceeding with other symptom categories. That being said, it is often helpful to begin with a symptom that has some meaning or that causes disruption for the child or youth, and that is not the most overwhelming to address. Early success breeds engagement and later success!

- *Triggers.* What are the triggers for the OCD-related distress/anxiety? These can be either external triggers (e.g., contaminated objects, proximity to a church, being near specific people, holding sharp knives) or internal triggers, which are the bodily sensations or obsessional thoughts themselves.

- *Core fears.* What are the core OCD-related fears? In other words, what are the "bad things" the child or youth believes will happen if they do not engage in a ritual? For example, some children with contamination obsessions have fears of getting sick or dying, some have fears of making others sick, and yet others fear that the associated feelings of disgust or distress will never go away. It is not sufficient to establish that a child is distressed by touching a doorknob. The clinician needs to know what the child thinks will happen if they come into contact with that doorknob. Younger children may have a harder time articulating these fears and may need clinician support to identify them. Specifically, they may fear that when something is not "just right," they will never lose their feeling of discomfort or distress.

- *Neutralizing the core fear.* How does the child or youth neutralize the core fear? In other words, what do they do (compulsions) or avoid to prevent the feared outcome? For some children, this will be easily apparent (e.g., checking compulsions, washing rituals, confessing). For others, the rituals may be more covert, either because they are engaging in mental rituals or they are purposely trying to conceal their rituals from others' observation. To develop effective ERPs, clinicians need to know specific details about the nature of the rituals so that they can be targeted for prevention following exposures.

- *Avoidance.* What is the child or youth avoiding? Many will engage in significant avoidance of obsessional triggers to prevent themselves from "having" to conduct rituals. For example, a child may use a barrier such as a shirt sleeve, tissue, or glove when touching objects that they fear are contaminated, to ensure they do not subsequently have to perform lengthy washing rituals. Identifying the specific objects, people, situations, or activities that are being avoided is key in developing an effective treatment plan. In fact, these answers often provide a wealth of ideas for future ERP exercises, as they can be used as exposure stimuli.

- *Family accommodation to OCD.* How are family members (and others) accommodating the child's or youth's OCD? In actuality, almost all families engage in some degree of accommodation of the child's OCD (whether they realize it or not!). ERPs cannot be effective if family members continue to accommodate the child's associated avoidances or compulsions. A later section in this book describes how to help families identify and then limit their accommodation. It is helpful before starting treatment to know how family members and potentially others (e.g., teachers, friends) accommodate OCD-related demands.

Obstacles to Treatment

Are there specific obstacles to treatment that need to be addressed? In addition to parental accommodation, many other variables can impact a child's or youth's progress in treatment.

These can include parents' own ability to tolerate their child's distress, parental psychopathology, and psychiatric comorbidities. Busy schedules and a resistance to adjusting them may prevent children and youth from devoting 30 to 60 minutes per day to practicing ERPs. A clinician cannot be expected to identify and address all possible treatment-interfering behaviors or variables prior to treatment, but an awareness of their potential to impact treatment is very helpful in guiding the treatment course.

OCD-Related Coercive and Disruptive Behavior

In recent years, increasing attention has been paid to the important roles of coercive and disruptive behaviors and rage in pediatric OCD as obstacles to treatment success (Lebowitz, Omer, & Leckman, 2011). While traditionally these had been highlighted in discussion of tic disorders, their emergence in the context of anxiety disorders and OCD had been underrecognized. Rage attacks are relatively common among children and youth with OCD and contribute to family accommodation, which can further affect the severity of symptoms and overall impairment (Stewart, 2012). Previously, many children demonstrating these types of extreme reactions in the context of OCD triggers were diagnosed as having comorbid oppositional defiant disorder (ODD) or conduct disorder (CD). Neuroimaging studies of OCD have added to the revised understanding of this illness, suggesting that increased emotional reactivity may actually reflect a failure of the higher-order parts of the brain (e.g., the dorsal frontal cortex) to exert control over the more primitive brain structures such as the amygdala (De Wit et al., 2015).

In many instances, OCD-affected youth have a history of being people pleasers and overachievers in academics, sports, and social realms. Parents are often shocked and confounded when their previously compliant child swears at them or throws objects at walls in the middle of an OCD-related episode. This may particularly emerge when the child is trying to avoid exposure to an OCD trigger, or when they face interference in ritual completion (e.g., parents refusing to provide reassurance for the 10th time). Module 4 discusses how to prepare parents to limit accommodations. For greater detail on addressing OCD and anxiety-related aggression, the book *Treating Childhood and Adolescent Anxiety: A Guide for Caregivers* (Lebowitz & Omer, 2013) describes the SPACE program (Supportive Parenting for Anxious Childhood Emotions) (see also Lebowitz, Omer, Hermes, & Scahill, 2014).

Pretreatment Ratings and Measuring Success

Predicting, encouraging and praising success are important components in the ERP process and along the path to beating OCD. Compared to the time frame for some other disorders that respond quickly to treatment, awaiting OCD response to treatment may require more patience.

For better or for worse, human beings adjust to and become desensitized to positive and negative factors in their lives. Children, youth, and family members who have suffered under the controlling and often longstanding influence of OCD may have limited insight into the depths of its negative effects. As such, it may be challenging for them to (1) believe that a different reality is possible; (2) understand the extent of OCD pathology, and family accommodation, and (3) recognize small changes and improvements when they occur.

As such, it is helpful to capture measures of OCD severity and its impacts at the start of treatment and throughout the treatment course. Clinician, parent, and youth measures are available to identify the frequently differing perspectives on illness and change. For the practicing clinician, open-source scales that are user friendly and free of charge are more practical than those requiring calculations or expense.

The following validated measures are available online and without cost on the International OCD Foundation website (*https://iocdf.org*):

OCD Symptom Types, Severity, Functional Impact, and General Improvement

- **CY-BOCS**—Children's Yale–Brown Obsessive Compulsive Scale (Scahill et al., 1997)
  - Clinician, parent, and child reports
  - 10 items + extension questions
  - Each item rated between 0 (none) and 4 (maximum)
  - Total severity score range (for 10 items): 0–40 (lower score = *better*)
- **CY-BOC-CL**—Children's Yale–Brown Obsessive Compulsive Checklist (Scahill et al., 1997)
  - Clinician, parent, and child reports
  - Items for OCD symptoms experienced in past week and ever
  - Obsession category symptoms (10 contamination, 3 somatic, 11 aggressive, 3 religious/moral, 4 sexual, 1 magical, 1 hoarding, 1 symmetry, 10 miscellaneous)
  - Compulsion category symptoms (5 cleaning, 1 superstition, 3 ordering/arranging, 8 checking, 3 repeating, 2 hoarding, 1 counting, 1 involving others, 12 miscellaneous)
- **COIS**—Child OCD Impact Scale (Piacentini, Peris, Bergman, Chang, & Jaffer, 2010)
  - 33 items
  - Each item rated between 0 (not at all) and 3 (very much)
  - Total score range: 0–99 (lower score = *better*)
- **CGI-S**—Clinical Global Impression Severity Scale (Guy, 1997)
  - Clinician, child, and parent versions
  - Single item
  - 7-point scale from 1 (no illness) to 7 (extremely severe symptoms) (lower score = *better*)
- **CGI-I**—Clinical Global Impression Improvement Scale (Guy, 1976)
  - Single item
  - 7-point scale from 1 (very much improved) to 7 (very much worse) (lower score = *better*)

Family-Related OCD Measures

- **FAS**—Family Accommodation Scale (Flessner et al., 2011)
  - Parent report
  - 12 items

- Each item rated between 0 (not at all *or* N/A) and 4 (extreme)
- Total score range: 0–48 (lower score = *better*)
- Subscales: avoidance of triggers, involvement in compulsions
- **OFF**—OCD Family Function Scale Part 1 (parent and child report) (Stewart et al., 2011)
  - 21 items
  - Each item rated between 0 (never) and 3 (daily/always), for both "current OCD" and "worst ever OCD"
  - Total score range: 0–63 (lower score = *better*)
  - Subscales: daily routine, social, work/school and emotional impacts
- **PT-CD**—Parent Tolerance of Their Child's Distress (modified from the Distress Tolerance Scale [Simons & Gaher, 2005])
  - Parent report
  - 15 items
  - Each item rated between 1 (strongly disagree) and 5 (strongly agree)
  - Total score range: 15–75 (higher score = *better*)
  - Subscales: tolerance, absorption, appraisal, and regulation

Other OCD-Related Behaviors

- **CD-POC**—Coercive and Disruptive Behavior Scale for Pediatric OCD (Lebowitz et al., 2011)
  - Parent report
  - 18 items
  - Each item rated between 0 (never) and 4 (almost all the time)
  - Total score range: 0–72 (lower score = *better*)

Intentional planning for regular measurement collection is recommended. While this may depend on individual circumstances, capturing scores at baseline and every subsequent six sessions is a reasonable frequency. This may help the child, parents, and even clinicians to recognize unappreciated gains and progress, in addition to unidentified persisting areas of OCD-related difficulty.

Pretreatment Checklist

For clinicians who are new to treating pediatric OCD, it can seem daunting to gather all the necessary information before starting treatment. The following checklist is meant to help clinicians track their readiness to start ERPs with a family:

- ☐ Is the child or youth engaging in any maladaptive coping skills (e.g., self-harm, substance use) that should be addressed first before starting ERPs?
- ☐ Have I assessed the potential impact of comorbidities on ERP outcomes? Should they be addressed before starting ERPs? For example, will the child or youth's

symptoms of depression (low motivation, low energy, and poor concentration) make it difficult to engage in ERP?

☐ Does the child or youth and family have the motivation to engage in treatment and complete daily ERPs? If not, are there some motivational interviewing strategies that should be implemented first?

☐ Do I have sufficient rapport with the child or youth and family to facilitate engagement in treatment?

☐ Have I explained what OCD is and how ERP works?

☐ Have I identified incentives that can be used as rewards for in-session and between-session ERPs?

☐ Does the child or youth and family have available time to set aside 30–60 minutes each day for ERPs? If not, are there changes that the family is willing to make to prioritize treatment?

☐ Have I imparted realistic hope to both the child or youth and parents about the possibility for change? Have I told the family that with hard work, we can realistically anticipate success for this child or youth? (See Chapter 1.)

CHAPTER 3

Fine-Tuning ERP Delivery

While the previous chapter provides details on planning CBT treatment for pediatric OCD, the following pages offer guidance and examples to help "fine-tune" CBT with respect to ERP management based upon OCD symptom type, age group, family factors, and treatment setting characteristics.

Fine-Tuning by OCD Symptom Type

The use of exposures in treating OCD can take two forms, *in vivo* and imaginal. The following presents examples of each and discusses which forms of exposure may work best with which OCD symptom types.

When to Use *In Vivo* Exposures

In vivo (i.e., "in life") exposures involve confronting obsessional triggers (e.g., situations, objects, images, or thoughts) in real life. Doing so allows the child or youth to habituate to distress-provoking stimuli while realizing that the feared outcome is unlikely to happen, or that it can be tolerated. Common examples of obsessions and related *in vivo* exposures are listed below:

- *Contamination obsessions:* contact with "contaminated" people, objects, or places without subsequent handwashing, or use of hand sanitizer or other forms of disinfectant.
- *Arranging/ordering obsessions:* leaving objects at school or at home in the "wrong" order or position without correcting them.

- *Uncertainty:* checking locks, stove, hair straighteners, etc., only once and resisting the urge to check again when near the trigger.
- *"Not-right" feelings:* engaging only once in an activity that provokes the "not-right" feeling and resisting the urge to perform an action that would "correct" the concern.

When to Use Imaginal Exposures

Imaginal exposures involve confronting fears or distressing situations in the imagination. Some feared outcomes are impractical or even impossible to re-create in real life. For example, it is not ethically (or legally) appropriate to simulate a situation in which another person is in actual serious danger. Similarly, some future feared outcomes cannot be realistically simulated, such as fears of going to hell. In these instances, it is useful to focus or bring to mind the feared situation and outcome for an extended period of time, with a goal of promoting habituation or fear extinction. Examples of obsessions that are suited to imaginal exposures are listed below:

- *Transformational obsessions:* fears of taking on the characteristics of specific individuals, or of losing aspects of one's own personality.
- *Religious obsessions:* fears of going to hell or of a deity being angry at them.
- *Sexual obsessions:* fears of sexual contact with taboo individuals, excessive doubt about one's own sexuality
- *Harm-related obsessions:* fears of harming oneself or others

Imaginal exposures involve purposefully focusing on distressing thoughts until habituating to them. With practice, the individual is able to experience these same thoughts without the extent of related distress or discomfort. With *in-vivo* exposures, the child or youth habituates to feared situations and objects. With imaginal exposures, the child or youth habituates to distress-provoking thoughts. See Module 5 for more information on conducting imaginal exposures.

Examples of *In Vivo* Exposures

The following pages describe many sample ERPs to help therapists in developing a specific treatment plan. These are intended to be general starter ideas and will require modification based on individual symptom presentation. It is also important to consider the timing of exposures in treatment planning. A good treatment plan involves creating an OCD Ladder (see Module 2), which can be used to develop and implement exposure activities.

Contamination Obsessions

- Rub candies on various "contaminated" surfaces (e.g., doorknobs, shoe soles, carpet, toilet seat) and then eat them.
- Rub an article of clothing on a "contaminated" surface and then wear it.

- Use a contamination rag. This involves rubbing a cloth or piece of fabric on a contaminated surface. After each instance of showering/hand washing/use of hand sanitizer, children or youth then recontaminate themselves by rubbing the cloth on their hands and body. The purpose of this activity is to reduce the sense of relief created by the washing compulsion. Don't forget to get them to "recontaminate" the rag as needed.
- Increase the degree of contact with "contaminated" objects. Start with a few fingers, then work up to a whole hand, then rub that hand over their face and body.
- To address excessive and/or ritualized handwashing, set limits on the length of washing time, amount of soap used, and how the washing ritual is completed. Consider implementing a washing or soap "holiday," whereby the use of washing (of any kind) or the use of soap is eliminated for a set period of time. Note: This is very hard for children and youth (and their parents) to attempt but can be extremely useful in many cases.

Harm-Related Obsessions and Avoidance

- Holding knives, scissors, and other triggering objects with increasing proximity to self or others. For example, if a child or youth is worried about harming a parent, have them work toward holding a knife against the neck of a parent. If they are worried about harming themselves, have them work up to holding a knife toward their own wrist.
- For fears of stealing items from stores, have the child or youth walk into a store and hold an item close to their backpack or pocket.
- For fears of being responsible for something terrible happening (e.g., starting a fire), turn on all the burners on the stove and leave the room, then work up to leaving the house.

Sexual Obsessions

- For children who have ego-dystonic doubts about their sexual orientation, have them look at images of peers of the concerning gender and say, "Maybe I like him, maybe I don't. I'll never know for sure."
- For children who experience distressing thoughts about being gay (e.g., "I just looked at that guy's butt. I must be gay"), have them comment on physical attributes of peers of the concerning gender. For example, have them look at friends on Facebook and say, "My friend John is really hot."
- For children who are afraid of acting on ego-dystonic aggressive sexual impulses (e.g., rape, pedophilia), have them spend time in triggering environments, like playgrounds. Have them repeatedly say or sing words in session that they have previously avoided (e.g., *sex, penis, vagina*).

Fear of Losing Things

- Have the child or youth leave a valued possession in a public place (e.g., iPhone, backpack) slowly increasing how public the location is and how long the child is away from the item.

Magical Thoughts and Superstitious Obsessions

- Have the child or youth perform activities in multiples of their unlucky numbers.
- Go outside and step on as many cracks as possible. This could be extended later to include walking on the sidewalk without monitoring steps so that it is unknown whether a crack has been stepped on.

Somatic Obsessions

- Have the child or youth research various diseases such as cancer or AIDS. Prepare a research project on the topic.
- Visit various clinics or hospital wards or even waiting rooms. Meetings with physicians can be helpful as well as long as they have been trained to not provide reassurance.
- For children or youth who fear vomiting, exposures to vomit and vomiting are key. These can involve looking at pictures of vomit, drawing pictures of vomit, watching YouTube videos of people vomiting, making fake vomit (minestrone soup works great), and pretending to vomit with it while saying "I feel so sick." For kids and youth who fear the physical sensations related to being ill, eating lots of candy then jumping on trampolines or spinning around can be a good way to create interoceptive exposures to nausea.

Religious Obsessions

- Hold the Bible while saying blasphemous thoughts. This can be made increasingly difficult by varying the location of the exposures. You can start by doing exposures in your office, then moving to areas near churches or other places of worship, and then eventually going inside these buildings.
- Drinking milk while staring at a meat product, if the individual has concerns they are not observing dietary laws of Judaism.
- Praying for bad things to happen.

Fine-Tuning by Age Group

A common fallacy is that ERPs cannot be conducted with young children. Many therapists shy away from working with young children. However, OCD is just as treatable at younger ages as it is at older ages—in fact it may be even more so as behavior patterns and parental accommodations tend to be less entrenched. This section will address how to adapt treatment for younger children.

It can sometimes be challenging to distinguish OCD behaviors from those indicative of normal developmental stages. Young children very often display ritualistic behaviors as a normal and important part of development. These behaviors typically emerge around age 2 and peak in the preschool years. For example, it is common for preschoolers to want to wear and do the same thing every day, arrange their favorite toys like cars in a certain way until they feel "right," and have elaborate good-bye or nighttime rituals before bed. Similarly, magical thinking is common in young children, including superstitious behaviors such as not stepping on cracks on the sidewalk. These factors present a challenge in determining whether to diagnose or treat OCD in young children. If magical thinking and ritualistic behavior are common to a stage of typical development, how then does one distinguish between normative development and pathology that would prompt intervention? A fairly simple approach can be taken when making this decision. If a child's thoughts and behaviors are causing significant impairment and interfering in their functioning or that of their family members, intervention is likely warranted.

When treating young children with OCD, parents serve as the main agents of change. Consequently, therapy *must* involve parents and typically parents are involved in all aspects of treatment. Some sessions may be conducted with parents alone and others jointly with the parent(s) and child, but it is almost never warranted that a session be conducted with the young child alone.

The key component of successful OCD treatment is exposure to triggering agents. This is no different when working with young children. However, OCD-focused CBT for younger children *must* be done in a more playful and fun way in order to keep them engaged. A key to this is finding out the child's interests and capitalizing on them when creating exposures. For example, when treating a little girl who likes the story "The Paper Bag Princess," the child can be asked to draw a picture of their OCD as a dragon and to draw herself as the princess who will make OCD go away with her magic wand. Children who like superheroes can be given a cape to wear and challenged to fight back again the evil OCD villain with their imagined superpowers. Once the time comes to create specific exposures, these themes can be used to keep the child engaged and to make it fun!

The following are key principles to observe when working with younger OCD-affected children:

- *Involve the parent.* A parent should be involved throughout the entire session with young children. This will allow modeling of the exposures they will do with their children at home. Accommodations can also be directly addressed in session through role-play activities.

- *Develop a reward system.* Take time to develop a good reward system. With younger children, rewards must be immediate and tangible, as it is difficult for them to defer gratification and postponed reinforcement will be less effective. Using candy with this age group can be particularly effective. For bigger prizes that they are working toward, it is beneficial to print out a picture of the prize, cut it into puzzle pieces, and have the child earn pieces of the puzzle for exposure practice. This gives them a concrete view of the progress they are making toward earning the prize.

- *Use age-appropriate strategies.* Have children draw pictures of the OCD as a meanie, monster, dragon, or other identified foe, and themselves as a superhero, princess, or other powerful protagonist. Get them to generate powerful, empowering statements to resist

OCD-related urges, such as "Go away, meanie—I don't have to do what you say . . . I'm the boss!" Practice in session saying these statements in an assertive voice while engaging in exposures.

- *Use images or sayings for fear ratings.* Do not get hung up on identifying exact fear ratings as young children will have difficulties generating numbers as indicators of their fear level. Use graphical illustrations of emotional faces as anchors, or expressions such as "You bet!," "Maybe," and "No way" to measure how much distress is expected before selecting exposures. Other forms of measurement include getting children to use their arms to measure fear or even rating anxiety as "small," "medium," or "big." If even these fear ratings are too challenging for the kids to identify, and if they are willing engage in an exposure, then follow their choice and craft each subsequent exposure to be slightly harder than the last. Fear hierarchies play less of a role and are often unnecessary with young children.

- *Make exposures fun.* Make all exposures fun and game-like to keep children engaged. (See Part II, Module 4, on ERP games.)

Fine-Tuning by Treatment Setting Characteristics

Technology-Based CBT

By reading this book, you as a clinician are taking steps to join the relatively small group of therapists knowledgeable about the gold-standard treatment for pediatric OCD. Specialized treatment such as ERP for OCD requires considerable skills that many do not possess, yet these skills are highly rewarding once obtained. Given that OCD is underreported, many generalist clinicians in rural areas may not identify enough cases to develop and hone these CBT skills. Access to evidence-based CBT for OCD is therefore challenging for many families to obtain. As such, recent efforts have been directed toward the use of technology to decrease the current gap in services.

Use of web-camera-delivered, family-based CBT, including ERP, has been investigated and has garnered support (Storch et al., 2011). By using computers and the Internet, many more families can access treatment. There are ethical issues around confidentiality and consent that are unique to this situation. Clinicians must ensure that the family understands the limits of confidentiality and security that may be present depending on the type of Internet platform being used (e.g., Skype, FaceTime, telehealth systems). It is also important to check with specific licensing boards to ensure coverage in the jurisdictions in which you are practicing and the one where the family lives.

Group CBT

The "OCD Is Not the Boss of Me" program as generally described in this book has been delivered via a family-based group format at the British Columbia Children's Hospital Provincial OCD Program since 2011. Many clinicians do not work with a sufficient number of

OCD-affected children and adolescents to warrant a group-based approach. However, a brief summary of a typical group session is provided below to illustrate how the 10 modules can be adapted for group therapy. Groups typically consist of up to six children or youth (ages 8–12 or 13–18) with at least two group facilitators and are 90 minutes in length.

1. After children or youth arrive for the group, therapists briefly check in with each individual regarding assigned ERPs and other homework tasks.
2. Each individual is asked to share with the group one of their assigned ERP activities from the week, which are charted on a board or flip chart. They are asked about progress with the ERP (i.e., if their anxiety or distress decreased over the course of the week when engaging in the ERP), how they managed to get through the ERP (e.g., coping self-talk, rewards), and how they can make the ERP more challenging for the next week. The purpose of this activity is twofold: (1) having the child talk in front of peers about their OCD and ERPs normalizes the experience of having OCD; and (2) having each child listen to others describe their symptoms and ERPs promotes generalization and consolidation of gains, as children are exposed to a wide variety of symptom presentations and related ERPs.
3. Play an ERP game (see the games described in Module 4).
4. Introduce a new topic or activity from the current module. Youth are encouraged to take turns reading and discussing the topic and are provided with opportunities to apply the strategy to their own OCD symptoms.
5. Spend most of the session practicing ERPs. Depending on symptom presentations of group members, children and/or youth can pair up or work in small groups to complete ERPs together.
6. Spend the final 15 minutes of each group session with parents and the child or youth together, and model for the parents how to be supportive yet firm and encouraging during ERP. Work individually with each family to develop ERPs to practice over the next week, and spend time problem solving around any treatment-interfering behaviors or other obstacles to treatment progress.

While therapists are working with children and youth in the treatment group, a concurrent parent group is run. This group allows parents to learn strategies similar to their children's so they can support ERP efforts at home. This group also allows parents to focus on parent- and family-specific topics, such as limiting family accommodations, addressing the impact of OCD on the functioning of the family, and parental self-care.

An outcome study was conducted of the "OCD Is Not the Boss of Me" family-based group approach, comprising 12 weekly sessions with separate child, youth and parent groups running concurrently for 90 minutes. We found that youth and families experienced significant decreases in symptom severity, functional impairment, coercive–disruptive behaviors, family accommodation, and family impairment by the end of treatment, which were maintained 1 month after completion of treatment (Selles et al., 2018a). We also found that coercive and disruptive behavior improvement mediated treatment response (Schuberth et al., 2018).

Intensive and Residential CBT

As noted previously, not all OCD responds successfully to CBT conducted on an outpatient basis, even by experienced clinicians. One of the many factors involved in CBT success relates to the frequency and intensity of treatment sessions.

During summer months since 2012, the "OCD Is Not the Boss of Me" manual formed the basis of an intensive family-based CBT group. Known as "Camp Oh-See-Dee," it provides 12 sessions over a 1-month period (rather than a 12-week period) and integrates camp-like games and activities into programming (McKenney, 2012). While the captured efficacy of the intensive and weekly forms of the program have been equivalent overall, the increased session frequency has been especially beneficial for specific families. For example, those who have difficulty ensuring homework completion at weekly intervals and those with poor distress tolerance requiring therapist encouragement and motivational influence have done particularly well in Camp Oh-See-Dee. A study by Storch et al. similarly found equivalent efficacy for CBT that was provided to groups with intensive (i.e., multiple sessions over 1–2 weeks) versus weekly frequency in pediatric OCD (Storch et al., 2007b). This supports the notion that success can be achieved in a shorter overall time frame. However, it appears that some individuals in the intensive group make greater gains with the higher frequency of sessions than that which would occur in the weekly format.

Residential treatment is another means of providing CBT. It is appropriate for individuals who have been unable to succeed with lower-frequency sessions, or whose OCD interferes with the most basic of daily functions or the ability to make it to sessions (e.g., morning checking and washing rituals lasting for several hours before leaving the house). There are unfortunately relatively few residential pediatric OCD treatment programs, and most are adult focused. ERP exercises are typically run for 2–4 hours daily in these programs, with other skill-building groups focused on mood regulation and coping skills to contribute to overall quality of life. While participants in residential treatment are typically affected by severe, debilitating, and complex OCD, adult studies have demonstrated their effectiveness in adults, and preliminary evidence supports their effectiveness in children.

CHAPTER 4

Complementary Approaches to ERP

In addition to the ERP techniques that comprise the main focus of this book, several complementary and augmenting approaches may selectively be used for pediatric OCD, depending on individual circumstances. This chapter describes these treatments, including primarily cognitive approaches, acceptance and commitment therapy (ACT), medication, and somatic treatments. Some of these are strongly supported by the literature (e.g., serotonin reuptake inhibitor medications; see Ivarsson et al., 2015), whereas others either lack evidence for use in pediatric OCD (e.g., ACT) or should only be used selectively and cautiously in conjunction with ERP (e.g., relaxation therapy, which is inferior to CBT and equal to placebo in decreasing overall OCD severity; Westwell-Roper & Stewart, 2018).

Primarily Cognitive Approaches

As noted in Chapter 1, the emphasis of "OCD Is Not the Boss of Me" is on ERP activities. However, if children or youth resist engaging in ERPs, therapists can start with behavioral experiments. Behavioral experiments can be conducted between or during sessions and involve gathering evidence that supports or refutes a child's beliefs. One version is the use of anonymous surveys regarding normative behaviors. Imagine working with an adolescent who experiences intrusive sexual thoughts and they believe that having such thoughts means they are a deviant individual and that such thoughts are not normal. An approach is to work together to construct a brief survey that asks the youth's peers to anonymously report their experiences with similar thoughts. The results are then reviewed and can be used to challenge the youth's beliefs that these thoughts are abnormal and that "normal" people don't have thoughts like this. Another type of behavioral experiment could involve asking questions of various experts. For example, if a child has many somatic complaints and worries that they are indicative of a serious medical condition, then the child could present a list of symptoms to a physician and ask whether any of these symptoms could also be caused by anxiety. In addition, a more active approach involves experiments where the child or youth does not engage in a safety behavior, predicts what will happen, and then compares this to what really happens. It is important to remember that this is not an ERP activity and that the purpose is not for the child to habituate to the obsessional trigger (although that can be an unexpected bonus!). Rather, the purpose is to gather evidence that challenges OCD beliefs as an adjunct to engaging in ERPs.

Some OCD symptom presentations and cognitive styles are more amenable to cognitive approaches, including overestimation of risk and overvalued sense of responsibility. That said, the use of cognitive approaches does not preclude the use of ERPs, as exposure-based approaches should remain a primary therapeutic tool. Use of the cognitive techniques described in this section will depend on the age and cognitive abilities of the child.

Inflated Responsibility

Inflated responsibility is one of the most common faulty cognitions involved in OCD. It refers to the belief that one has power to bring about or prevent negative events from occurring. This is often seen in individuals with harm-related obsessions and related compulsions (e.g., "If I don't make sure the stove is off, there could be a house fire").

The use of a *responsibility pie chart* can be a helpful way for youth to recognize their tendency to take responsibility for events that are beyond their control. The process begins by asking the child to identify a negative outcome that they feel responsible for and assigning a rating for how responsible they feel for causing that outcome to occur (e.g., 80%). Consider the following example:

> Mark believes that if he doesn't say his goodbye ritual to his mother before she leaves for work, then she will be injured or killed in a car accident during her morning commute. He believes that he is 100% responsible for keeping his mother safe.

Mark is asked to generate a list of other possible contributors to the negative outcome that are unrelated to his actions. In the illustrated example, the following possible causal factors for car accidents are identified:

- Poor weather/road conditions
- Distracted drivers on the road
- Mechanical problems
- Inexperienced drivers

He is then asked to assign a percentage of responsibility for each contributor to the event occurring, with the total equal to 100% or less. If Mark's mother was involved in a car accident what percentage of that outcome could be attributed to poor weather and road conditions? Distracted drivers on the road? The therapist helps Mark to plot these on a pie chart (Figure 4.1), being sure to leave any remaining nonassigned portion of the pie to himself.

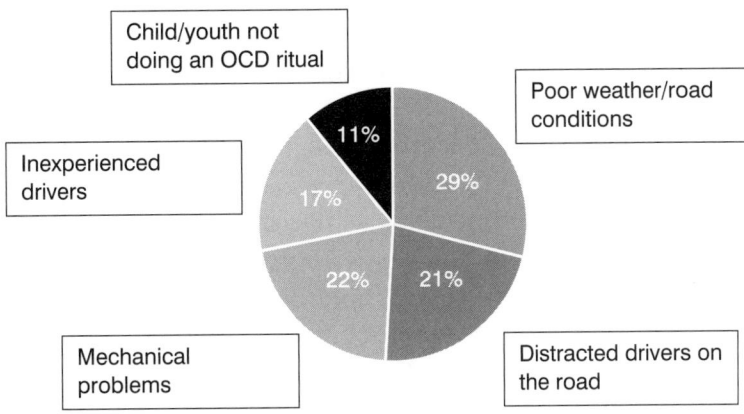

FIGURE 4.1. Mark's responsibility pie chart.

The therapist can then compare the youth's original estimate of responsibility to what remains as their contribution in the pie chart. The purpose of this activity is not to absolve children such as Mark of responsibility (although the exercise can result in nothing being left in the pie chart for the youth); rather, this activity is designed to highlight OCD's tendency to make children feel responsible for things that are outside of their control, and to demonstrate that multiple factors contribute to outcomes (both positive and negative). OCD is simplifying matters by assigning responsibility to the child and their rituals. The goal of this exercise is to highlight the difference between perceived and actual responsibility, rather than the percentage of responsibility itself. It is not helpful for the child to then focus on what is left ("But I'm still 11% responsible for keeping my mom from having a car accident"). Therapists must also be careful that the conclusion from this exercise is not to provide the child with reassurance that they are not at all responsible. Instead, the goal is for the child to recognize that they tend to feel overly responsible for events. Receiving reinforcement via reassurance is a risk of any cognitive exercise, which is why cognitive activities should be followed by a series of ERP tasks that target the uncertainty. In the case of this specific example, a series of ERPs could include having the child complete the ritual incorrectly or shorten the ritual and then ride out the subsequent anxiety.

Overestimation of Threat

Another common cognitive error that can perpetuate OCD is the tendency to overestimate the perceived threat associated with intrusive thoughts. The probability calculator, which is based on the work of Van Oppen and Arntz (1994), is designed to address an individual's tendency to overestimate the likelihood of a negative event occurring. It begins by having the individual estimate the probability of their feared outcome occurring. Consider the following example:

> Samantha is a 17-year-old girl who is worried that she will contract a serious illness if she comes into contact with a homeless person. OCD is making her believe that there is a 10% chance of this happening.

The therapist and Samantha generate the sequence of events that would have to transpire for this feared outcome to occur, and Samantha then estimates the probability of each step in the sequence (see Figure 4.2).

The therapist then helps Samantha to calculate the cumulative probability of all these events occurring. In other words, the probability percentages of all the events in the sequence occurring are multiplied together. This allows for the comparison of the perceived chance of the single feared outcome (contracting an illness from a homeless person) to the chance that each occurrence in the chain of events will culminate in the feared outcome. This allows Samantha to realize that her estimated probability of getting sick from a homeless person (10%) is significantly inflated compared to the cumulative chance that she will get sick from a chain of events that begins with a homeless person speaking to her (0.00001%).

The purpose of this exercise is not to prove to Samantha the irrational or extremely low likelihood of the event occurring. Focusing on the low probability of the feared outcome only serves as a form of reassurance and undermines the treatment plan. For many children and youth, focusing on the probability itself will reinforce the risk ("There is still a 0.00001% chance of getting sick. I can't take even that small chance, so I must keep avoiding homeless people"). Rather, the aim of this activity is to illustrate that the individual may have a tendency to overestimate the risk of the feared outcome. This realization can help prepare them for subsequent ERP activities in which they are exposed to obsessional triggers and subsequently resist urges to engage in rituals, avoid the threat, or neutralize their fears in some way.

Cognitive strategies should typically not be used in isolation. In other words, once the child or youth is able to acknowledge that they are making faulty estimates about the likelihood of a negative event occurring, then the therapist follows up with ERPs. Cognitive strategies are designed to help recognize and acknowledge faulty beliefs, not to trigger arguments about the actual likelihood that the feared outcome could come true. Subsequent ERPs will help children to realize that they can tolerate the uncertainty about whether the feared outcome will come true.

Acceptance and Commitment Therapy

For some youth, engaging in systematic and consistent practice of ERPs does not result in habituation to their intrusive thoughts. For such individuals, including aspects of ACT into the ERP therapy program may be recommended. Although ACT and ERPs both fall under

Event	Probability
1. A homeless person speaks to her.	20%
2. That particular homeless person has a communicable disease.	25%
3. As he speaks, a drop of saliva lands on her.	18%
4. Her hand then brushes against that part of her body.	15%
5. The droplet of saliva is transferred to her hand.	8%
6. The next time she eats, the droplet gets into her mouth, thereby infecting her.	10%

FIGURE 4.2. Samantha's probability estimates.

the umbrella of CBT, there are a few fundamental differences that set ACT apart from ERPs. ACT is more focused on shifting the way our inner experiences, including obsessions, are experienced as they are considered part of our lives. Rather than trying to directly target obsessions, ACT helps children find a way to diminish the impact of obsessions and anxiety on their lives, so even if obsessions remain intense and time-consuming, they can lead a meaningful life that is consistent with their values and goals. ACT aims to keep individuals engaged in a wide range of value-driven behaviors after experiencing intrusive thoughts, rather than being restricted to specific compulsions. In other words, children continue to live their lives and engage in activities that are meaningful to them (e.g., homework, spending time with friends) despite experiencing obsessions.

The use of ACT for OCD is relatively new and research on its effectiveness is still emerging (Twohig, Whittal, Cox, & Gunter, 2010; Twohig et al., 2018). ERP remains the first-line treatment approach, but incorporating ACT into treatment may be beneficial in situations when habituation does not occur during ERPs or when the youth is unable or unwilling to attempt ERPs. A comprehensive description of ACT is beyond the scope of this book. Readers interested in learning more about ACT with adolescent clients are directed to the book, *ACT for Adolescents: Treating Teens and Adolescents in Individual and Group Therapy* (Turrell & Bell, 2016).

Relaxation Training: Benefits, Risks, and Appropriate Use

Physiological symptoms of anxiety can be managed through relaxation exercises, such as diaphragmatic breathing, progressive muscle relaxation (PMR), or guided imagery. These are excellent tools for managing stress and anxiety outside of the therapeutic ERP context; however, there is growing consensus that relaxation therapy may be contraindicated in the treatment of anxiety disorders, as well as OCD. There are several reasons for this:

1. Dampening the experience of anxiety during exposure activities may interfere with the process of habituation, in that the child may not have the experience of anxiety decreasing on its own (i.e., "getting used to it").
2. If a child utilizes a relaxation technique whenever they feel anxious, they lose the opportunity to learn that they are able to withstand this sensation.
3. The relaxation exercise can become a new compulsion or "escape behavior."

That being said, it can be helpful to teach children and youth various relaxation techniques to manage general life stress. This is because the severity of numerous illnesses (including OCD, tics, hair pulling, skin picking, and other disorders) tends to worsen during times of increased stress. Relaxation skills can also be encouraged in specific contexts. It is important to provide very clear guidelines as to when one should and should not use these strategies with regards to OCD symptoms. The guidelines are as follows:

- When practicing ERP activities, do *not* encourage use of relaxation strategies during response prevention. Emphasize riding out the distress such that habituation or tolerance are enabled to occur.
- For unexpected anxiety-provoking, OCD-triggering situations in which the urge to

do a ritual is perceived as impossible to resist, use relaxation strategies as a nonoptimal but preferred alternative to rituals.

The need for selective use of relaxation methods in OCD management cannot be overemphasized, as families often present with a treatment history including relaxation strategies (but not ERP or CBT), and a stated goal of "getting rid of" thoughts that make the child or youth anxious. Empirical evidence is clear that relaxation strategies alone are *no better than placebo* in treating OCD. In other words, it is not possible to "deep breathe" your way out of OCD. In fact, encouraging this approach within certain contexts may be detrimental. It is important that the family does not interpret the message as "anxiety is bad and needs to be eliminated" instead of the preferred message, "Even if I am anxious, I am strong enough to deal with it—it might be my brain or my OCD tricking me—I shouldn't pay attention to it, even though it's trying to get my attention."

Before introducing relaxation strategies, it is important for the child or youth to have an awareness of how anxiety feels physiologically in their body. It can be helpful to draw an outline of a person and have them draw their experiences in the figure (e.g., butterflies in the stomach).

One of the most effective relaxation tools is diaphragmatic breathing (commonly referred to as deep breathing, balloon breathing, or belly breathing). Children tend to favor deep breathing over other strategies such as progressive muscle relaxation and guided imagery because it can be performed anytime, anywhere, and without anyone else observing it. And as above, it can be very useful during times of stress, while struggling to fall asleep, or when confronted with a real-life OCD trigger and resisting a ritual does not seem possible.

There are several points to convey when teaching children or youth deep-breathing skills:

- The breath should go in through the nose and out through the mouth.
- As the child inhales, they should notice their belly expand, like a balloon filling with air, while the chest and shoulders remain still. The breathing needs to be slow—fast breathing is hyperventilation and will actually increase the feeling of anxiety (due to low carbon dioxide levels in your blood).
- The exhale should be longer than the inhale.
- The skill must be learned and practiced when the child or youth is relaxed in order for it to be readily available to use during more anxious and stressful times.
- Encourage at least 10 cycles of breathing to see the benefits—both during practice and during the real thing!

Keeping the above points in mind, the following are some favorite ways to teach deep breathing. Choose one that fits the developmental level of the child or youth.

- *Blowing bubbles.* Using bubbles can help younger children with their breathing. It incorporates the same principles described above but uses bubbles to make the experience more fun!

- *Stuffies go up the hill and down the hill.* Using the child's favorite stuffed animal or "stuffie," have them lie down flat on the ground on their back. Show them how to expand their stomach by breathing in through their nose so their stuffie goes "up the hill" and explain that when they let the breath out through their mouth, the stuffie goes "down the hill."

- *Balloon breathing.* Have the children imagine a balloon in their stomach. Have them place one hand below their belly button. Instruct them to breathe in slowly and deeply through their nose to a count of four, feeling the balloon fill up with air. When the balloon is full, have them breathe out slowly through their mouth, to the count of five or six to deflate the balloon.

- *Smell the roses/blow out the birthday candles.* Have children imagine that they are holding a rose and smelling it really slowly and then have them imagine they are slowly blowing out a birthday candle.

- *Smell the pizza and then cool it off to eat!* Along similar lines, some children like the idea of imagining themselves smelling a slice of pizza and then blowing on it to take a bite.

- *Box breathing.* The last technique, which works well for older children and teens, is called box breathing. In this technique, have the youth imagine the four sides of a box. Have them draw the box in the air with their index finger. Breathe in for four (up one side of the box), hold for four (across the top of the box), breathe out for four (down the other side of the box), and wait for four (across the bottom of the box).

After trying out one or several of the above, have the child or youth brainstorm other types of activities that can help with relaxing (e.g., listening to music, going for a walk, taking a bath). Also ask them to come up with ideas for when and where they can practice their deep breathing when they are not feeling stressed. Finally, help the child or youth to generate the times when they might use deep breathing (e.g., going to sleep, taking a big test), and other times when it is not a good idea to use it (e.g., during ERPs). Doing this will also ensure they understand how important it is to *not* use relaxation strategies while doing exposures.

Medication and Somatic Approaches

Medications

As described in Chapter 1, OCD is fortunately a disorder with proven treatment approaches. The most important of these in pediatric OCD is CBT, specifically that which incorporates ERP. However, each OCD-affected individual is unique, and response may be suboptimal, requiring use of alternate or augmenting approaches. With respect to preferences related to first-line treatments, approximately 55% of OCD-affected adults prefer ERP while 45%

prefer SSRIs (Patel, Galfavy, Kimeldorf, Dixon, & Simpson, 2017). With respect to augmentation of SSRI treatment for OCD, ERP is notably preferred over antipsychotic medication (68% and 31%; $p < .001$). Preferences of OCD-affected children and youth and their families have not yet been studied.

When to Consider Medications

For specific OCD-affected children and youth, medications can play an important role by establishing necessary, and otherwise difficult-to-achieve, conditions for ERP success. These may include individuals with high OCD severity, poor insight, low motivation, interfering comorbid conditions, or lack of access to qualified ERP clinicians with OCD expertise.

When OCD is moderate or severe, bossing back OCD may appear to be impossible for a child or youth, a challenge akin to climbing Mount Everest. The goal of medication use in these instances is to decrease the intensity of OCD-related distress to a point where success is imaginable, shrinking the perceived journey to a challenging but achievable and rewarding hike up a steep hill.

In other circumstances, comorbid diagnoses or symptoms may interfere with chances for ERP success. For example, lack of motivation, low energy, and cognitive slowing associated with depression may be targeted with an antidepressant. Conveniently, first-line OCD medications are also identified as antidepressants. Extreme distractibility and hyperactivity associated with ADHD may also be targeted via medication, with the goal of improving engagement in ERP. However, in some cases stimulants may be poorly tolerated prior to OCD management due to worsening of anxiety as a side effect.

While combining CBT with medications appears to lead to improved results (70% response, 53% remission) versus those achieved via medications alone (42–50% response, 21% remission), debate remains about whether this combination is superior to CBT alone (62% response, 39% remission; POTS Team, 2004; O'Kearney, 2007; O'Kearney, Gibson, Christensen, & Griffiths, 2006). Nonetheless, in individual situations where OCD is at least moderately severe and CBT gains have been limited, an OCD medication trial is worth consideration.

Specific OCD Medications

As noted in Chapter 1, serotonergic reuptake inhibitors comprise the only clearly proven treatment approach for pediatric OCD other than CBT. These first-line medications include SSRIs and the tricyclic antidepressant (TCA) clomipramine. While children or youth may respond to one individual SSRI more than another, findings indicate that none are superior in treating groups of OCD-affected children (Geller et al., 2003). Overall, and similar to adult response rates, approximately one-half of OCD-affected children and youth will respond to a first SSRI trial (Bloch & Storch, 2015).

Given the above suboptimal response rates, it is at times necessary to augment SSRIs or clomipramine in the treatment of OCD. Atypical antipsychotics have been demonstrated as moderately effective augmenting agents in adult OCD (NNT = 5), and especially for individuals with comorbid tics (who also have poorer response to SSRIs; Bloch et al., 2006). In contrast to dose and duration of SRIs for OCD, doses of augmenting agents are relatively low and most studies have been of short duration (see Table 4.1). Unfortunately, alternative medication strategies have not been well studied in treatment-refractory pediatric OCD. In adults, potentially beneficial approaches other than antipsychotic augmentation include raising SSRI dosage and the addition of glutamate-modulating agents such as memantine (Bloch & Storch, 2015).

Specific Challenges Arising in Medication Use for Pediatric OCD

Child, youth, and parent factors may contribute to unwillingness to attempt an OCD medication trial. One of these factors relates to symptoms of OCD itself, such as concerns about contamination via ingestion of "chemicals" or the need for certainty around OCD diagnosis. This may interfere with the child or youth's openness to taking a medication.

Unlike parental decisions to accept a bronchodilator trial for their asthmatic child, or a steroid trial for their youth with juvenile arthritis, parents too often face guilt and criticism when considering whether to begin an OCD medication trial for their child. They may fear unknown harm to their child's brain, uncertainty about the emergence of side effects, or associated stigma and shame. Some parents may have a belief that OCD is a product of poor parenting or other factors, without a biological basis, or that the child should earn their improvement via CBT.

Stigma and fear of side effects are two main reasons for family hesitation regarding OCD medications. In addition, lack of clinician familiarity with higher SSRI dosages and

TABLE 4.1. OCD Medications

Generic name	Trade name	FDA approved for OCD (age)	Starting dose (mg/day) Child	Starting dose (mg/day) Teen	Target dose (mg/day) Child	Target dose (mg/day) Teen
SSRIs						
Citalopram	Celexa	n/a	2.5–10	10	20–40	40
Escitalopram	Lexapro/Cipralex	Adult	2.5–5	5	10–20	20
Fluoxetine	Prozac	7 years+	2.5–10	10–20	40–80	80
Fluvoxamine	Luvox	7 years+	12.5–25	25–50	200–300	300
Paroxetine	Paxil	Adult	2.5–10	10–20	40–60	60
Sertraline	Zoloft	6 years+	12.5–25	25–50	100–200	200
TCA						
Clomipramine	Anafranil	10 years+	25	25	Variable	
Augmenting medications (added to SSRIs or clomipramine)						
Risperidone	Risperdal	n/a	0.25–0.5[a]	0.25–0.5[a]	0.25–1.0	0.5–2[a]
Aripiprazole						

[a]Decrease risperidone dose by half if using in conjunction with fluoxetine or paroxetine.

longer trials (compared to those more commonly used for anxiety and depression) may lead to unnecessarily slow dose escalation or premature and inappropriate discontinuation in pediatric OCD. Prior to concluding that an SSRI is ineffective, a 10- to 12-week trial with 3 weeks at the target dose (or highest tolerated dose within range) should be attempted (Geller & March, 2012).

Adverse Effects

Unfortunately, SSRI side effects tend to emerge prior to beneficial OCD response, which may take 10–12 weeks. While adverse effects tend to be inconvenient rather than dangerous, they may be especially challenging for the very young and for those with health-related obsessions. SSRI-related gastrointestinal symptoms such as stomach upset, diarrhea, and constipation often self-resolve after a few days once serotonin receptors in the gut adjust to the medication, and insomnia or sedation are often managed by changing dose timing.

Behavioral effects including agitation, irritability, and disinhibition are less likely to self-resolve and more common in younger children, emerging after 4–6 weeks and with increased doses. In addition, risk of cardiac arrhythmia dictates that a maximum citalopram dose of 40 mg be used.

"Black-box" warnings regarding potential risk of suicidality with antidepressant use in children can be very concerning for parents and clinicians. However, reanalysis of the data by diagnoses (Bridge et al., 2007) suggests the suicidality difference between SSRI (number needed to harm [NNH] = 200, NNT = 6 in OCD) and placebo (0.5% absolute risk difference) is lower in OCD than in depression (NNH = 112, NNT = 10).

Given the above, best clinical practice indicates that discussions with youth and families are required to set realistic expectations prior to beginning a medication trial. This includes the following points:

- Time of full trial at a high dose (10–12 weeks).
- Required dose (high end of range).
- Potential side effects (cost–benefit).
- Counteracting effects of drugs/alcohol, comorbidities, etc.
- Preference to pair meds with CBT.
- Adherence.
- Planned discontinuation and tapering (if desired) following 6- to 12-month stability.
- Imparting of hope.
- Measurement of change (via CY-BOCS and other scales).

Transcranial Magnetic Stimulation and Deep Brain Stimulation

Invasive approaches studied in adult OCD include repetitive transcranial magnetic stimulation (rTMS) and deep brain stimulation (DBS). However, these have not been well studied in pediatric OCD or with respect to impacts on neurodevelopment, mandating caution. The few rTMS studies conducted to date suggest that brain activation may be a promising approach in adult OCD (De Wit et al., 2015).

DBS is a U.S. Food and Drug Administration (FDA)–approved treatment of adult OCD that involves placement of an implantable pulse generator within specific brain regions (Naesström, Blomstedt, & Bodlund, 2016). Follow-up data on six adults with OCD indicated that DBS of the ventral capsule/ventral striatum region was safe and conferred long-term symptom reduction benefits in OCD but not depression (Fayad et al., 2016). However, this has not been well studied in pediatric OCD, a group with distinct ethical considerations.

PANDAS/PANS Management

As noted above, PANDAS/PANS treatment approaches are not well defined by empirical evidence. A common misperception by families is that the standard pediatric OCD treatment approaches of CBT and SSRI/clomipramine are ineffective for PANDAS/PANS. While a recommendation has been made to introduce medications more slowly and by smaller dose increments in these putative subtypes, there is no evidence of ineffectiveness of standard medication approaches in these situations. Moreover, given the intensity of symptom presentation and family impairment, particular attention in CBT should be paid to limiting accommodation and appropriate management of rage and disruptive behaviors.

Given the putative autoimmune/inflammatory role, it has been postulated by some that a helpful approach to take is to minimize pro-inflammatory response (via daily omega-3 fatty acids with EPA > DHA), to maximize barriers to infection (probiotics to strengthen the gut microbiome), and to promptly treat infections (i.e., with appropriate antibiotics). The role of long-term prophylactic antibiotics is unclear, with studies to date reporting divergent results (Sigra, Hesselmark, & Bejerot, 2018).

Further discussion of this topic is beyond the scope of this book. However, interested readers are directed to respected websites such as that of the International OCD Foundation (*https://iocdf.org*).

PART II
Providing Treatment
10 Nuts-and-Bolts Modules

Each module in Part II follows a similar format. We provide you with detailed information about various aspects to include in your treatment program, most of which are also included in the reproducible worksheets and handouts. Treatment sessions typically follow the plan below, though feel free to use your clinical judgment to tailor your sessions to each child's or youth's individual needs.

1. Review.
    a. Successes and challenges with assigned home practice (e.g., ERPs, symptom monitoring, developing a reward program).
    b. Therapist Update worksheet completed by parents (included with each treatment module).
2. Introduce new module/continue with module from last session (as needed).
3. In-session ERP (preferably with parent observation of some ERPs).
4. Plan for between-session ERP practice.
5. Review of session and wrap-up.

We try to include parents in as much of the session as possible, with parents present for the entire session when children are 10 years old or younger. Adolescents may prefer that parents be less involved in sessions. In such situations, we typically have parents join for the initial part of the session to review progress to date and problem-solve around identified challenges, and then have them rejoin the final portion of the session for a review of what was covered and to plan for between-session practice.

MODULE 1

Treatment Preparation with the Child or Youth and Their Parents

Education about OCD and Orientation to Treatment

Education plays an essential role in the treatment of OCD. In treatment, children, youth, and their parents will be asked to engage in activities that are often challenging and intrinsically aversive. Children and their parents may also have misinformation about OCD, and it is important to correct any misunderstandings so that everyone is on the same page!

There are four main components to include in psychoeducation:

1. Explaining what OCD is, including clarification of obsessions versus compulsions, and introducing the goal of stopping compulsions but not necessarily eliminating obsessions (i.e., we cannot control our thoughts, only our actions).
2. Externalizing OCD as separate from the child's or youth's identity such that the child, family, and clinician can ally as a team against it.
3. Recognizing that OCD behavior varies across time and settings—differences do not indicate that the symptoms are "faked," or that one parent's home is "better" than the other.
4. Explaining how treatment works, especially the rationale for ERPs.
5. Describing expected outcome for treatment and building motivation.

Explaining OCD

The first component to explain is what OCD is and how it works. This explanation will vary depending on the age and developmental level of the child. In the "OCD Is Not the Boss of Me" program, OCD is referred to as a bully in the child's head; it's trying to get the child to do things they wouldn't otherwise want to do. We use this because the concept of bullies is highly relatable to school-age children and teens. With younger kids, it can be explained that OCD is like a meanie or a monster trying to get them to do things they don't want to do. Here is a specific example of how to explain this:

> "Bullies like attention. If they pick on a kid, and the kid cries or gets mad, the bully gets what he wants, and becomes a little bit more powerful. And so, he comes back for more. Sometimes it's really hard to stand up to a bully. Sometimes you need to get an adult to help. The OCD bully is the same. When you do what the OCD bully wants you to do (like wash your hands, check the locks, arrange things a certain way, or whatever else your OCD bully tells you to do), the OCD gets a little bit stronger. The bully comes back for more and more. It's really hard to stop the OCD bully on your own. Adults you trust can help. Your parents and I will be part of your team to help you to boss back the OCD bully."

Adolescents will benefit from a more sophisticated approach from parents and clinicians about OCD and the treatment approach. We like to capitalize on adolescents' desire for independence and their resistance to being controlled by focusing on OCD's ability to get teens to do things they don't want to do (i.e., compulsions) and make them think things that upset them (i.e., obsessions). Here is a specific example of how to talk to teens about OCD:

> "OCD is really messing things up for you. It's this voice in your head that you can't ignore that is tricking you into doing things over and over again that you don't want to do and that you know don't make sense. OCD won't let you focus on what's important, like school and friends. Instead, the OCD is trying to control your thoughts and won't let you move on. This means you're spending way too much of your time paying attention to OCD and doing what OCD wants and not enough time doing what you want. It's really hard to push back against OCD, but your parents and I want to work with you so that you're the one in control, and not OCD."

Differentiating between Obsessions and Compulsions

It is important to help children and youth distinguish between obsessions and compulsions. Often children, youth (and adults!) mix these two up. This distinction becomes important when exposures begin, given that it is the obsessions and triggers that children are exposed to. These contrast with the compulsions and behaviors, which are targets of change that will be eliminated. An example of how to clarify the difference between obsessions and compulsions is as follows:

> "Have you ever tried to watch TV but couldn't change the channel? It usually means that the batteries in your remote control are dead. When this happens, you can't change the channel to get to your favorite cartoon. Instead, all you can watch is the news or a scary movie. OCD works the same way. It's like you can't change the channel from the

upsetting thoughts that the OCD bully wants you to be stuck thinking about. When you get stuck on a bad thought that is upsetting to you, it's called an obsession.

"Obsessions are unwanted and upsetting thoughts, images or ideas that get stuck. They're different from regular worries about real-life issues, like homework or fights between friends. Obsessions keep coming back, over and over again. You don't want to be thinking these things, and you can't control them. You've probably tried to get rid of the thoughts; you've ignored them, or distracted yourself, but they end up coming back. Obsessions take up a lot of energy and they make it hard to focus on homework, enjoy your downtime, or even spend time with friends doing activities or sports that you usually enjoy.

"Compulsions are also called rituals and are different from obsessions. Compulsions are actions, like habits that you do over and over to prevent something bad from happening or to make the obsessions and bad feeling go away . . . and this works, for a little while. This is why you do it again. But the more you do the compulsions, the stronger the urge is to do them again in the future. It's like the bully who keeps coming back for more. You do what he says to make him go away, but he only goes away for a little while. Over time, you end up giving in and doing more and different compulsions to make the OCD bully go away. Kids with OCD often don't want to do these things, but they feel like they have to anyway."

It is a good idea to have kids and youth generate lists of obsessions and compulsions at this point to solidify these concepts, and to assist in later creation of a "map" of the areas to be targeted with exposures.

Externalizing the OCD

OCD has a way of causing a lot of conflict in the home, drawing family members into fights with each other. Because of this, it is important to focus everyone's energy on one enemy: OCD! By externalizing the OCD, a common language can be established. Sometimes it is helpful to lay it out in terms of teams: Team OCD versus Team Child. Externalizing the OCD can be done in different ways depending on the age of the child. Younger children can be asked to give OCD a name and to draw a picture or create their OCD out of clay. Older children and teens often prefer to call it by its proper name of OCD. The exact chosen name matters less than the process of identifying OCD as a target that is separate from the child's or youth's identity. Here is an example of how this conversation could be started:

"Let's draw a picture of what your OCD Bully looks like and give it a name so we know who we're dealing with. This is who we're going to start bossing back. Examples from other children who I've worked with include 'Mr. Clean,' 'The Doubter, and 'The Germinator.' You can also just call it 'OCD' if you like."

Here are some simple ways to modify language that will help the child (and parents) to see OCD as something outside of the child:

- "The OCD bully is being really bossy right now."
- "What is the OCD bully making you worry about?"
- "The OCD bully is making you wash your hands too much. We don't have to listen to him."
- "The OCD bully wants you to avoid touching that. We're going to do the opposite of what the bully wants."

Externalizing the OCD serves two purposes. First, it allows the child or youth, parents, and therapist to unite together against a common enemy. It sends the message that everyone is on the same team and committed and motivated to fight back against OCD. Second, it allows children, youth, and families to think differently about the child's symptoms and their impact on the functioning of the family. Rather than being blamed for engaging in behaviors that others feel they should be able to control, family members come to see their child (and themselves) as victims of the OCD bully, who need support and encouragement, rather than blame or ridicule.

Explaining How Treatment Works, Especially the Rationale for ERP

Start by explaining that there are generally two main types of treatment for OCD: CBT and medications. It will be important to explain that ERP is a specific type of CBT. The process of setting up an exposure is explained in detail in Module 2. Refer to that module in order to provide a detailed explanation of ERP exercises. Below is a starting explanation for how treatment works:

> "Research on OCD has shown that there are two helpful types of treatment: cognitive-behavioral therapy (CBT), which is what you'll be doing here, and medication. Both of them lead to brain changes that can actually be seen in brain scans called MRIs. CBT teaches kids and youth new ways to think about and react to the thoughts and urges that come with OCD. It gives you the tools you need to fight the OCD bully. With CBT, kids learn to face their worries and resist OCD-related behaviors and urges. Some kids may also take medications for their OCD, which can make it easier to be successful."

What Are ERPs?

The main component to explain to the child and parents at this point is that ERP is the best weapon in the fight against OCD. Study after research study has clearly shown that ERP is the active ingredient in successful CBT for OCD. The following provides a simplified explanation of ERP and how it works. You will have an opportunity to discuss this in more detail with families in Module 2.

> "ERP is just a fancy way of saying 'facing your fears.' Specifically, it involves exposing you to the trigger, situation, object, image, thought, or idea that typically makes you

feel anxious, scared, grossed out, disgusted, or really uncomfortable. Then, in response prevention you ride out the uncomfortable feeling and resist the compulsion."

Describing the Expected Outcome for Treatment: Inspiring Hope

It is important to communicate that with hard work, this therapy works! You want to set up a realistic expectation for success. It is also helpful to tell families that the more they put into this treatment, the more they are likely to get out of it. As mentioned previously, families should be asked to set aside 30 to 60 minutes per day to practice fighting back against OCD. This often involves a commitment to cut back on some other activities while in therapy. At this point, remind the family about how much time OCD is taking up now in their daily lives and which will likely increase, which could be restored with successful treatment, making the investment of their time and best efforts very worthwhile. For example:

> "After successful treatment, most kids and teens have either gotten rid of their OCD or decreased its power over their lives. But the OCD bully can come back. The good news is that you're starting the process of learning how to manage your symptoms so that if and when an OCD thought creeps back in, you'll know what to do. With the help of your parents, your therapists, and this program, you can get control of your OCD symptoms starting today.
>
> "If you're like most kids and teens with OCD, you've been living with obsessions and compulsions for a while and they've taken up a lot of your time. OCD has stopped you from doing a lot of things you enjoy and has messed a lot of things up. You've probably even gone to a lot of trouble to avoid things in your life that tend to trigger your OCD. Well, with this treatment, we aim for you to get back that time in your everyday life, and for you to be able to do the things you used to before the OCD bully took over. So it will be important for us to do our best and spend the time needed to make you and your family strong against the OCD to drive it away."

It can be helpful to have children, youth, and their parents think of and write down the ways that OCD has negatively impacted the child and family—this activity can inspire hope by suggesting ways that life could be different and better once the child's OCD is under control.

Using the OCD Ruler to Rate Distress

One of the first tools that children and adolescents should be taught in treatment is how to monitor and gauge their own level of distress—be it feelings of disgust, anxiety, fear, or "not-right" feelings—using a rating traditionally referred to as subjective units of distress scale (or SUDs), which measures the intensity of an experienced negative emotion. In terms of OCD, this rating will be used to report how a child or youth is feeling when experiencing an intrusive thought or to report their level of distress when they are unable to perform a ritual in line with OCD's demands and "rules." SUDs can range from 0 to 100 or 0 to 10. When working with children and youth, it is often preferable to simplify the rating and use only 0 to 10, with 0 reflecting the child feeling at ease/no distress, and 10 reflecting the highest distress, discomfort, or anxiety a child has ever felt. This also forces a decision to settle upon an "imprecise" account, as individuals can struggle with reporting an exact, precise score that worsens with a larger range of potential "perfectly accurate" answers.

The "OCD Is Not the Boss of Me" program uses a concrete model of a ruler, which we call the *OCD Ruler*, to reinforce the concept that one is measuring a level of distress. This follows the tradition of the *Feelings Thermometer* used in Kendall's Coping Cat program (Kendall et al., 2005) and others. This tool is purposefully referred to as the "OCD Ruler," and not the "Anxiety Ruler," to reflect the fact that OCD triggers a variety of distressing emotions in children and youth, including disgust, fear, "not-right" feelings, and other types of discomfort.

When introducing the OCD Ruler, the therapist can ask the child or youth whether they have ever used a ruler and explain the purpose of the ruler. It is helpful with younger children to have a standard plastic or wooden ruler in session for them to hold and to practice measuring whether something is small, medium, or large in size. The child can subsequently be shown the picture of another ruler, the OCD Ruler, which is used to measure the size of their negative feelings. The OCD Ruler will be used at several points in treatment. Initially, the child or youth will use the ruler to rate the level of distress at various steps on the constructed hierarchy (Module 2). Later in treatment, they will use the ruler to rate the level of distress experienced during an ERP to reflect on the habituation process.

Following you will find a sample of how we would introduce the concept of the OCD Ruler to a child or youth in session.

Sample Dialogue

THERAPIST: So, Max, just like a ruler measures things, we can measure how upset your OCD makes you by using a ruler. Our ruler goes from 0 to 10. So let's practice a bit using a ruler to describe your feelings about non-OCD stuff that happens in your life. How worried, scared, or upset would you be if your teacher gave you a surprise quiz tomorrow in math class?

MAX: I guess around a 3 or 4. It wouldn't be horrible, but I think I would sure be a bit worried if I wasn't prepared.

THERAPIST: Okay, so how about if I gave you a big piece of chocolate cake right now?

MAX: That's silly, of course . . . I would be at a 0—who would be afraid of chocolate cake?

THERAPIST: Now– last practice question, what if a big tiger burst into this office and there was nowhere you could run to escape?

MAX: So easy– obviously it would be a 10 . . .

THERAPIST: Okay, so let's apply this to your OCD symptoms. How distressed would you feel if you saw . . . ?

While the OCD Ruler is typically a beneficial component of CBT, it is important to be aware of its limitations in specific circumstances. For some children, the nature of their OCD symptoms makes it difficult to provide ratings of distress. They may attribute meaning to specific numbers, such as good or bad luck, making it more (or less) likely that they will report certain numbers. For example, if a child or youth feels compelled to complete activities in a specific number of intervals, then they may feel they should pick that same number on the OCD Ruler to ensure good luck. Similarly, if a child associates a feared outcome with a specific number (e.g., 6 is associated with the devil), then they may avoid providing that rating in an OCD-inspired effort to ensure their safety or the safety of others.

For others, the excessive OCD-related doubt experienced around making decisions may render it extremely difficult to select any number. Those with "just-right" obsessions may perseverate on whether they are feeling a 6 or a 6.5, while those who are unable to tune in to their emotional experiences may be unable to differentiate between their experience of an 8 versus that of a 3.

If a child or youth's OCD symptoms make it difficult to provide ratings on the OCD Ruler, then consider using an alternative method to obtain this information. All children can typically provide ratings reflecting small, medium, and high distress. Alternatively, consider providing phrases that reflect different levels of distress, as follows:

- "No big deal. I got this." = 0–2 (minimal distress)
- "Okay, I'm feeling anxious, but I'll be able to cope with this. It's somewhat hard, but I'll get through this." = 3–6 (moderate distress)
- "Whoa. This is hard. I'm having trouble coping. I'm really uncomfortable. My body is telling me to run away. Sound the alarm!" = 7–10 (high distress)

For those who struggle to tune in to their own emotional experiences and who cannot decipher distress experienced at an 8 versus a 2, various physiological indicators may be used as a proxy for their feelings of distress, as follows:

- Slight muscle tension = minimal distress (minimal distress)
- Heart pounding/increased breath rate = high distress 7–10 (high distress)

For younger children, colors may be used to convey distress. Using the analogy of a traffic light, green = "Good to go," yellow = "Whoa, this is getting hard," and red = "Stop, this is too hard." Other children may prefer to use manipulatives, such as toys of different sizes or pictures of faces to reflect various intensities of distress.

In the end, the specific method of obtaining SUDs does not matter. What matters is that the child or youth has a way to indicate to the therapist, parents, and/or themselves their various degrees of distress. This provides a way to decide which ERPs to engage in at a particular time, and to measure how specific obsessions and their related compulsions are responding to treatment over time.

Monitoring Symptoms: Increasing Awareness of Obsessions and Compulsions

Another strategy that can be helpful early in treatment is having the child or youth monitor the frequency of obsessions and compulsions. Although not a key component of the treatment program, symptom monitoring can be helpful in increasing a child's awareness of how often they experience an intrusive thought and/or how often they engage in a ritual. For those children or youth who may minimize their OCD or who have low insight, monitoring symptoms can help youth recognize the severity of their OCD and the need for treatment. Symptom monitoring has other benefits as well, including informing parents about the severity of symptoms, as intrusive thoughts and mental rituals are not observable by others. As well, if monitoring reveals that there are days of the week where symptoms are experienced at a higher rate, therapists can explore with the youth specific patterns or triggers on those days, which can help inform the development of ERPs later on.

Encourage the child to select one obsession and one compulsion to track between sessions. The obsession and compulsion do not necessarily have to be connected. Ask the child to use the Catch the OCD Bully worksheet and chart how many times they experience a particular obsession and engage in a particular compulsion each day. For youth who spend an excessive amount of time completing a ritual (e.g., extended showers, lengthy nighttime prayers), have them track how long they spend engaging in the ritual. If youth are completing rituals dozens of times per day, ask them to track a selected ritual within a specific time frame (e.g., between 4:00 and 6:00 P.M.). Children can track symptoms as they experience them on the worksheet, or complete the tracking at the end of the day.

The point of this activity is to increase awareness of symptoms as a foundation for later treatment strategies. Use your clinical judgment about when and if to introduce this strategy, and how long the child should be monitoring symptoms. Typically, the authors have the youth monitor symptoms for the first few weeks of treatment, and then remove this expectation once the family is regularly completing ERPs.

Treatment Preparation with the Parents

As you begin engaging with the youth in treatment, it is equally important to prepare parents with respect to treatment goals and expectations for what they will be asked to do (and to refrain from doing) in the coming sessions. Regardless of OCD severity, history, and past treatment efforts or failures, it is crucial to exude optimism and confidence while clearly describing the tasks to come. Higher parent treatment expectations prior to CBT have been linked to better outcomes in OCD severity, impairment, homework, and treatment completion (Lewin, Peris, Lindsey Bergman, McCracken, & Piacentini, 2011).

Preparing the Parent for Their Role in Treatment

Given the impact that OCD has on family functioning, and the near certainty that each parent accommodates OCD in at least some aspects, it is important that parents are actively involved in the treatment process. When describing the treatment plan, stress the importance of family involvement to enable successful outcomes. It should be communicated that their child's OCD therapy sessions will require more from them than other parental tasks, such as carpooling to a soccer game or sending cookies for a school bake sale. In other words, parents should not expect to drop off their children, return 50 minutes later and continue on with the next errand on their list. Parents are to be involved in many aspects of treatment, such as offering support for their child's ERP attempts, limiting accommodations, implementing and reliably following through on a reward program, and sharing their observations about obsessional triggers and rituals with you as a therapist. Generally speaking, more active involvement of parents in sessions prepares them to be better equipped to help with out-of-session ERPs as appropriate. The ideal degree of parental involvement varies according to the child or youth's age, maturity level, symptom presentation, and degree of parent–child conflict and insight. Treatment works best in low-conflict, low-blame family settings when parents are closely aligned with their child or youth in the fight against OCD, whether it be through involvement in ERPs (e.g., to limit reassurance seeking) or by validating their child's struggles while messaging their confidence that the child can succeed in resisting OCD. Parental involvement also conveys to their child that the family is united against a common externalized enemy, which is OCD.

Example Script to Prepare Parents for ERP Treatment

"Based on work I've done with other families, I know how much OCD can impact almost everyone in the home. Parents often end up feeling stressed, helpless or guilty for being unable to help their child, or angry at being 'blackmailed' by the OCD behavior. Most often, they experience a combination of these emotions. Making things worse, a child's parents frequently experience contrasting emotions, which can lead to conflict and isolation at a time when they need each other's support as coparents (regardless of their status as a couple). Fighting OCD is difficult, especially when it has been around for a long period of time. It is tough both for the child and for the parents to live with OCD, and sometimes even harder to start to fight it so that it goes away.

"Because of this, it will be important for you to set aside time in the coming weeks to support your child's fight against OCD and to work on some of your own homework. Again, OCD often ends up bossing around parents—and it takes practice and repetition to figure out responses that do not support or feed the OCD, but that help to decrease your child's OCD behaviors. Even if you don't tend to get personally pulled into OCD behaviors, I will need your help to know how your child responds to ERPs, and how they seem to be functioning across all areas of their life as we go through the sessions ahead."

Externalizing OCD and Limiting Blame

Most parents experience anxiety, sadness, and frustration on an almost constant basis as a result of their child's OCD (Stewart et al., 2017). Externalizing the child's OCD is very important as it helps to safeguard and repair the OCD-induced damage inflicted upon child–parent and child–sibling relationships. Parents may feel as though they are betraying their child by knowingly allowing them to suffer. Externalizing the OCD allows parents to reframe their understanding of limit setting and accommodation. This becomes increasingly important as treatment progresses, particularly when families are asked to address longstanding patterns of accommodation. When parents start to resist OCD-related demands they may experience a number of emotions including anxiety, sadness, and frustration. Rather than viewing this as a denial of their child's requests and needs, parents are asked to view this resistance as denying OCD's demands, which will only strengthen its power over time without intervention. It also helps parents to deal with and express the feelings they are experiencing in a way that does not hold their child accountable.

Depending upon individual parent characteristics and personal history, observing one's child in a painful struggle with OCD may elicit diverse responses. Some parents become highly distraught and anxious themselves when observing their child in distress. This may drive efforts to remove their child's OCD-related suffering "at any cost" and as quickly as possible, or to prevent a repeat of such suffering in the future. Most commonly, this is manifested by acts of accommodation—even acts that defy reason or require great effort and sacrifice on the part of the family. This also explains why, despite being intelligent and informed about negative impacts of family accommodation on OCD outcomes, parents may continue to accommodate their child's OCD.

Parents also experience inevitable frustration and anger in many OCD scenarios. When triggered, children or youth may go to whatever extent necessary in order to get parents to meet the momentary demands of OCD. This may include accusations that if the parent "really loved them" they would help, or that the parent hates them and is angry at them. By externalizing the OCD, parents can be coached to reply with a statement such as "Yes, you're right. I am feeling angry right now—I am angry at the OCD for how hard it is making our lives and for how upset it is making you. I don't want to keep doing things that make it stronger. I know that we can beat the OCD bully together."

Clarifying the Parent's Role

Parents need to allow the child to take responsibility for and a leading role in their treatment. This is often very difficult for parents who are used to having more control over their child's activities, and for those with low tolerance of their child's distress, which tends to lead to accommodation and "rescue" behaviors. It may be helpful to convey the following messages to parents who struggle with limiting their overinvolvement in treatment:

- Parents cannot do the ERPs for their child. They can, however, offer support, encouragement, and rewards for their child's efforts to complete ERPs.
- Taking a step back is not the same as punishing your child or abandoning them to face the OCD on their own.
- Allowing your child to take responsibility for their treatment plan is a way of demonstrating your confidence in their ability.
- Given that OCD has the potential to recur, it is vital that your child learns how to manage their disorder independently.

So how can parents find the balance between being an active supporter versus being overly involved in treatment? It may be helpful to describe the various roles to the family through an analogy such as the following (can be adapted to fit individual situations):

> "Think about this fight against OCD like an NBA basketball game. You are on one side of the court, and OCD is on the other side. Every ERP is like a jump ball, with both teams fighting for control of the ball (which is your life). Your parents will be on the sidelines, cheering you on. Every time you get control of the ball, you're winning in the fight against OCD."

Parents as Cheerleaders and Reporters

One of the therapist's jobs is to "coach" or teach strategies that help the child or youth ride out their anxiety or distress via in-session ERPs, performed in ways that can generalize to ERP practice between sessions. The main role of parents in this process is that of cheerleaders—acknowledging when their child is struggling, praising their efforts, recognizing the progress that they've made, and demonstrating confidence in their child's abilities to eventually overcome OCD.

It is generally counterproductive for parents to assign themselves the role of "OCD police"—which could include nagging children about ERP homework completion and questioning whether every little behavior is an OCD symptom. Parents can nonetheless provide concrete support by removing obstacles that may interfere with ERP completion (e.g,. lack of time, obtaining required ERP objects that are not available in the home). However, if a child or youth consistently avoids ERP tasks, this is an issue best left to be managed by the therapist. Parents should be encouraged to inform the therapist about progress and challenges that occur between sessions. Thus, important roles of the parent include that of cheerleader (to improve the child's motivation and confidence to take on OCD) and of reporter (to assist the therapist in modifying and fine-tuning the treatment plan).

What Parents Should Avoid Doing

In addition to encouraging parents about what they should do with respect to ERPs, it is important to advise them on actions to avoid. Parents must be careful to not express their own anxiety, distress, or disgust while their children are completing ERP homework. This is frequently very challenging, as watching one's child experiencing and enduring strong negative emotions can trigger a "rescue response." Moreover, parents with OCD or OCD tendencies may be also triggered by the exposure itself. A helpful analogy for parents to consider is the situation of a pilot speaking over the intercom to passengers before going through a period of turbulence.

From a passenger's perspective, the following message is helpful as it is honest, confident and optimistic:

"Ladies and gentlemen, we will soon be passing through an area of turbulence. It will likely get a little bumpy, but we'll be through it soon enough. Sit back, keep your seat belts on, and enjoy the ride."

In contrast, passengers would likely be more distraught after listening to the following message:

"Ladies and gentlemen, hold on tight. We're soon going to be experiencing some serious turbulence. Whatever you do, don't get out of your seat. I have no idea when we'll get through this. I've never experienced turbulence like this in my 20 years of flying . . . Maybe we should turn around . . ."

In the above scenario, the child or youth is the passenger, the turbulence is the ERP, and the pilot is the parent. The message to parents is the need to model adaptive coping skills during their child's ERPs. Children look to their parents for subtle (or overt) cues as to how they should be feeling in an unfamiliar situation. A parent who exudes confidence in their child's ability to cope will be more likely to inspire in their child a willingness to take a risk and challenge the OCD. A parent who appears anxious or distraught about their child's ERP challenge will more likely inspire the child's resistance to facing their fears, which will undermine chances of treatment success.

Preparing Parents for Their Child's ERP-Related Distress

When beginning therapy with a family, it is a good idea to prepare both the parents and children for what is to come. It is best to be completely transparent by informing families that the journey they are about to embark on will not be easy, but that it will be very rewarding. Explain that exposures will incorporate as much fun as possible and rewards will play a big role. Nonetheless, be clear that exposures will be challenging and distressing at times. And these uncomfortable feelings are critical to the success of the treatment. The goal is for children to learn that being uncomfortable and experiencing distress is not a terrible or dangerous thing that must be remedied immediately. Families and parents need to be prepared to witness their child's distress and to tolerate it without trying to alleviate it or to rescue them in the moment. The parents should be informed that tolerating their child's short-term distress without reinforcing OCD will eventually lead to the end goal of the child functioning without the constraint and constant fear of triggering the OCD bully.

Parents are naturally hardwired with the drive to alleviate their children's distress. In OCD treatment, it is critical that parents go against this "natural" response and actively ignore the child's behavioral manifestations of distress (e.g., crying, screaming, whining, begging), while at the same time praising and celebrating brave coping behaviors and indications of distress tolerance (e.g., sticking with the exposure despite being upset). Parents may need some practice at tolerating distress, and they can be directed toward resources such as mindfulness skills training that might be helpful in this regard.

Self-Care for Parents

Parenting a child with OCD can be experienced as a tremendous burden, especially when it is unclear how to help the child while protecting the family from crisis. Additionally, the treatment of OCD requires significant time and emotional resources from parents, often at the expense of their own well-being. If parents have not been taking care of their own personal needs and have become run down, it will be very challenging for them to implement the techniques and changes being asked of them in bossing back OCD.

OCD can be draining on parents for a number of reasons:

- Children and youth may demand unrelenting parental reassurance.
- Parents are often directly involved in many of their child's specific rituals.
- Rituals often interfere with the parents' daily functioning, such that they are late for work or distracted during other life tasks.
- Bedtime and nighttime rituals can interfere with parents' own sleep.
- Parents often experience confusion and stress about how to manage and limit-set unwanted behaviors that may potentially be OCD-related.
- Parents may experience increased worry and anxiety about their child's well-being and their future potential given their OCD diagnosis.

In order to be an effective cheerleader in the child or youth's battle against OCD, it is vital that parents be aware of the toll OCD can take on their child and on themselves. Parents often report that they feel selfish for taking any small amount of time for themselves rather than focusing on their children. This sentiment is even more prominent in the case of parenting a child or youth who is ill with OCD. In fact, the nature of OCD makes it even more important that parents have access to their full energy and resources. The treatment of OCD requires a family approach, and it is important to explain to parents that they are going to need to draw on their reserves of energy in order to support their child effectively. They are more likely to remain patient, supportive, and able to tolerate their child's distress and limit accommodations when they are well rested and have put aside time for themselves. Anecdotally, parents often have a very hard time with this concept and need assistance in sorting out how to dedicate time each week to foster their own needs.

Homework Assignments

For Module 1, therapists can assign the following for youth and parents to complete at home before the next session:

For Youth
- Complete the Catch the OCD Bully worksheet (symptom monitoring).

For Parents

- Complete the Parent Monitoring worksheet (parent observations of various compulsions, avoidance behaviors, and accommodations that the child requires, as well as estimated per-day average of each, and how parents responded).
- Complete the Therapist Update worksheet. This worksheet allows parents to share with the child's therapist any new OCD symptoms that were observed over the week, any particularly challenging OCD situations the family encountered, any successes that the child experienced, and any other information parents feel would be helpful for the therapist to know. Therapists should ask parents to provide them with this completed worksheet at the start of the next session so they can address specific issues as needed with the child or with the whole family together.

MODULE 1 HANDOUTS AND WORKSHEETS FOR CHILDREN OR YOUTH

Welcome

Psst . . . hey you . . . yeah, you . . . wondering why you are here today? Well, you have something called OCD, "obsessive-compulsive disorder." But hey—you know that. You also know that this OCD thing is really messing up your life. It's keeping you from having fun with your friends. It's making everyone argue. It's stressing out your whole family. It's making school really hard. What you might not know is that you can get better! And that's why you are here today.

But first, what is this OCD thing anyway? OCD is a bully in your brain. It tries to boss you around and make you do things you don't want to do. In this program, you're going to learn how to boss back the OCD bully. You are going to learn to say, "OCD is not the boss of me!"

Let's draw a picture of what your OCD bully looks like and give it a name so we know who we're dealing with. This is who we're going to start bossing back. Examples from other children include "Mr. Clean," "The Doubter," and "The Germinator." You can also just call it "OCD" if you like.

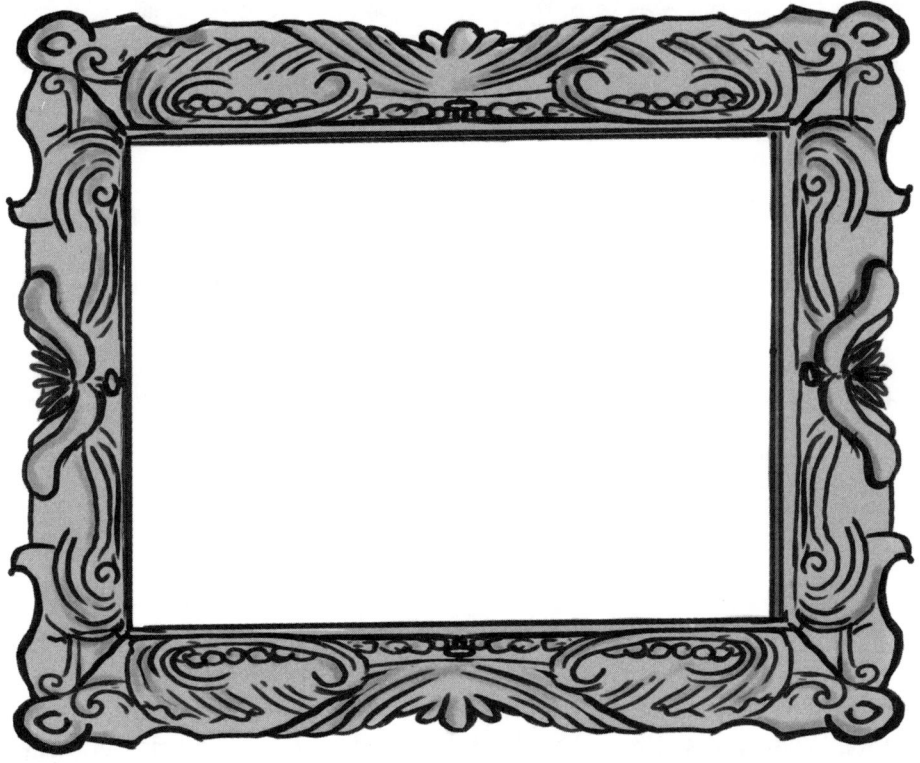

(page 1 of 8)

From *OCD in Children and Adolescents: The "OCD Is Not the Boss of Me" Manual* by Katherine McKenney, Annie Simpson, and S. Evelyn Stewart. Copyright © 2020 The Guilford Press. Permission to photocopy this material is granted to purchasers of this book for personal use or use with children or youth and their parents (see copyright page for details). Purchasers can download additional copies of this material, in color (see the box at the end of the table of contents).

Heroes are really good at fighting bullies. Who is your favorite hero? It could be a superhero, your mom, or anyone else you think is really brave. Draw a picture of your hero.

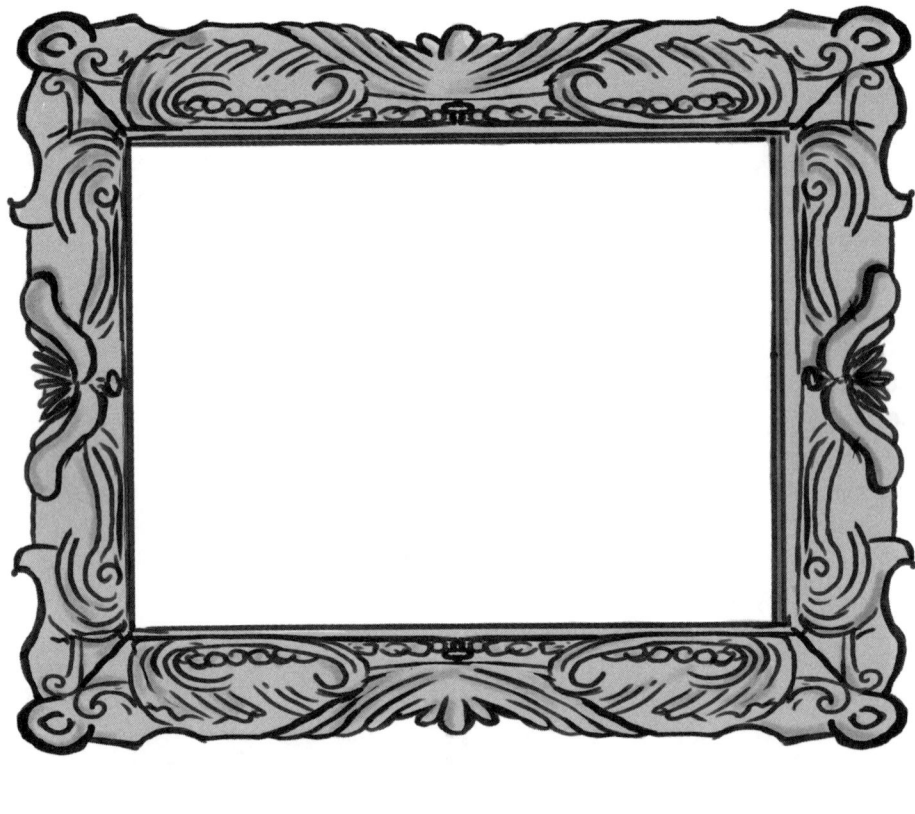

Your Hero

When you're learning how to boss back the OCD bully, think back to this hero to help yourself be brave.

Throughout this program, you're going to see small backpacks, like this:

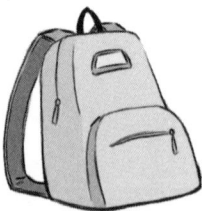

Each session you're going to learn a tip, trick, or "superpower" to help you boss back the OCD bully. When you see a backpack, it means that you're learning about a strategy that can help you fight the OCD. Not every strategy is going to work for every person or in every situation. You need to be able to pick and choose strategies from your backpack that work the best against your OCD bully.

(page 2 of 8)

You're also going to find blue thought bubbles, like this:

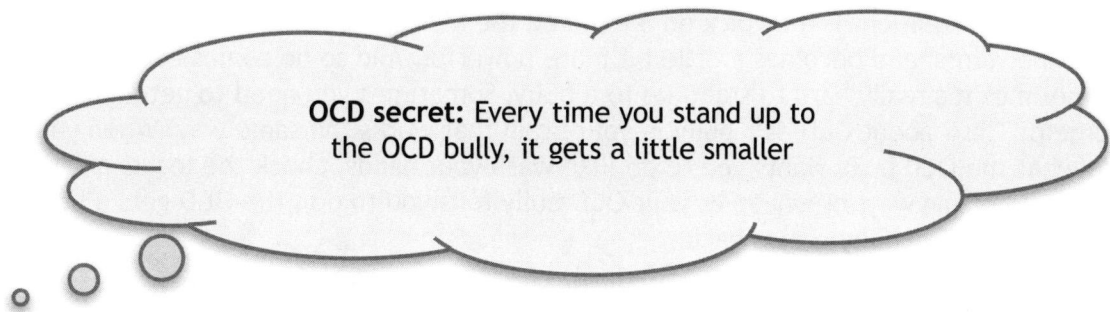

OCD secret: Every time you stand up to the OCD bully, it gets a little smaller

They are filled with secrets the OCD bully doesn't want you to know. Once you know the secrets, you can use them along with all the other tips and tricks in your backpack to boss back the OCD.

This program has two main goals:

1. To teach you about OCD.
2. To teach you strategies to manage your OCD.

What are your goals for the program?

_____

_____

_____

_____

_____

_____

_____

(page 3 of 8)

What Is OCD?

Bullies like attention. If they pick on a kid, and the kid cries or gets mad, the bully gets what he wants, and becomes a little bit more powerful. And so he comes back for more. Sometimes it's really hard to stand up to a bully. Sometimes you need to get an adult to help. Think about OCD as a bully in your brain that works the same way. When you do what the OCD bully wants you to do (like wash your hands, check the locks, arrange things a certain way, or whatever your OCD bully tells you to do), the OCD gets a little bit stronger. The bully comes back for more and more. It's really hard to stop the OCD bully on your own. Adults you trust can help. Your therapist and your parents will be part of your team to help you boss back the OCD bully.

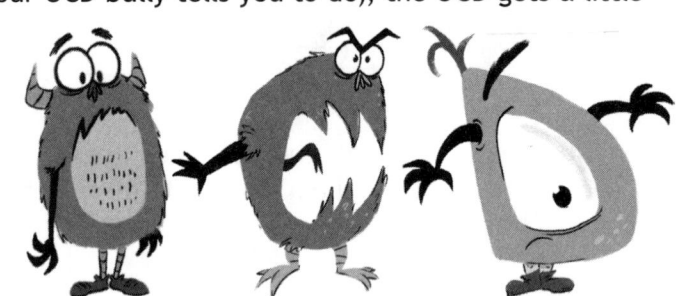

What Are Obsessions?

Have you ever tried to watch TV but you couldn't change the channel? It usually means the batteries in your remote control are dead. When this happens, you can't change the channel to get to your favourite cartoon. Instead all you can watch is the news or a scary movie. OCD works the same way. It's like you can't change the channel on the upsetting thoughts that the OCD bully wants you to think about. When you get stuck on a bad thought, it's called an obsession.

Obsessions are unwanted and upsetting thoughts or images or ideas that get stuck. Obsessions keep coming back over and over again. They're not just regular worries about real-life issues, like homework or fights between friends. You don't want to be thinking these things, and you can't control when they get stuck. You've probably tried to get rid of the thought, ignore it, or distract yourself but it doesn't work. Obsessions take up a lot of energy, and they make it hard to focus on homework, watch TV, or even spend time with friends.

Let's start by making a list of your obsessions so we know what we're dealing with:

_____

_____

_____

_____

What Are Compulsions?

Compulsions are behaviors or habits that you do over and over to prevent something bad from happening or to make the obsessions and anxiety go away . . . and it works, for a little while. But the more you do the compulsions, the stronger the urge is to do the rituals again in the future. It's like the bully who keeps coming back for more. You do what he says to make him go away, but he only goes away for a little while. Over time, you have to keep doing more and different compulsions to make the OCD bully go away. Kids with OCD don't want to do these things, but they feel like they have to anyway.

Let's make a list of your compulsions:

_____

_____

_____

_____

Why Do I Have OCD?

Unfortunately, we don't have a good answer to that question. We don't know why some kids get OCD and others don't. We do know that OCD tends to run in families. But even if you're the only member of your family with OCD, it's important to remember that you're not alone. OCD is about as common as diabetes in kids and there are probably other students at your school who also have OCD. It's also important for you and your parents to know that you didn't do anything wrong to get OCD—in other words—it's not your fault.

How Do You Treat OCD?

Studies on OCD have shown that there are two helpful types of treatment: cognitive-behavioral therapy (CBT), which is what you're doing in this program, and medication.

CBT teaches kids new ways to think about and react to the thoughts and urges that come with OCD. It gives you the tools you need to fight the OCD bully. With CBT, kids learn to face their worries, boss back OCD, and do the opposite of what OCD is telling them to do. The most important tool in CBT for treating OCD is called exposure and response prevention, or ERP. ERP is a fancy way of saying "face your fears." In ERPs, kids slowly expose themselves to things that make them feel anxious, gross, uncomfortable, or just "not right," and then they ride out the urge to do what OCD wants them to do, like wash their hands, check the locks, make things even, or do some other kind of ritual. We'll learn more about ERPs in the next session. Some kids may also take medications for their OCD, which makes it easier to stand up to the OCD bully.

(page 5 of 8)

Will It Go Away?

After successful treatment, most kids aren't bothered by their OCD symptoms anymore. But the OCD bully can come back. The good news is that you're starting the process of learning how to manage your symptoms so when an OCD thought creeps back in, you'll know what to do. With the help of your parents, your therapist, and this program, you can get control of your OCD symptoms starting today.

Why Get Rid of the OCD Bully?

If you're like most kids with OCD, you've been living with obsessions and compulsions for a while, and they've taken up a lot of your time. OCD stopped you from doing a lot of things you enjoy. You've probably even gone to a lot of trouble to avoid things that tend to trigger your OCD.

Make a list of all the ways OCD has messed things up for you:

_____

_____

_____

_____

The good news is that we're going to start changing things so OCD doesn't cause as many problems as before. Once we've got the OCD bully under control, you'll be able to do things you enjoy without as much stress or anxiety.

Make a list of things you'll be able to do once OCD is under control:

_____

_____

_____

_____

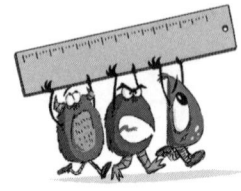 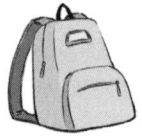

One of the first things we're going to learn is to measure how bothered you feel in different situations. We do this by using the **OCD Ruler**. It ranges from 0 (easy/not bothered) to 10 (too hard/out of control), and it will help us measure how upset you are in different OCD situations.

(page 6 of 8)

OCD RULER

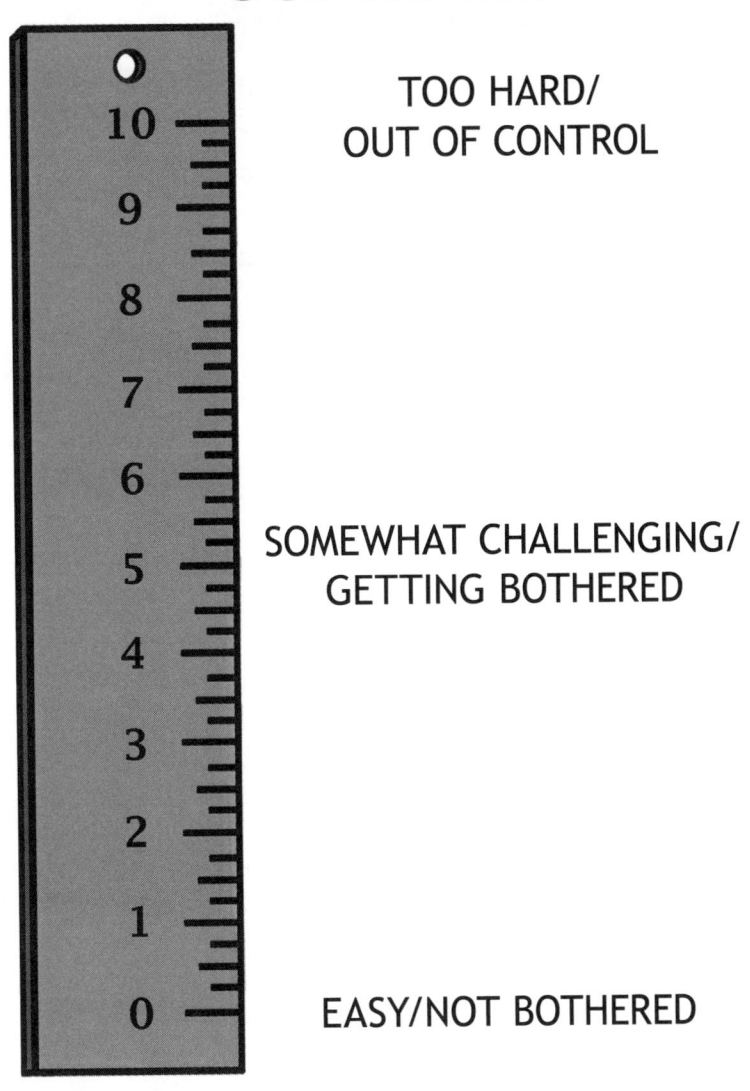

TOO HARD/
OUT OF CONTROL

SOMEWHAT CHALLENGING/
GETTING BOTHERED

EASY/NOT BOTHERED

Let's think about the different obsessions and compulsions that you have. We're going to write them down and rate them using the OCD Ruler. How bothered do you feel when you get stuck on an obsession or are unable to do a compulsion the way the OCD Bully wants?

Obsessions	OCD Ruler (0–10)	Compulsions	OCD Ruler (0–10)

We're not going to work on everything at once. We're also not going to start working on any that you rated as a 9 or 10. We want to start with OCD situations that are a little hard for you—but not awful!

Which ones do *you* want to start with? Look at your list and select a few obsessions and compulsions that you rated as 5 or lower. Circle them so we know what to start with.

Catch the OCD Bully

Before we can start bossing back the OCD bully we need to figure out where it likes to hide. We can do this by noticing how often you get stuck on an obsession or have to do a compulsion each day. This session pick one obsession and one compulsion to keep track of on your *Catch the OCD Bully* worksheet.

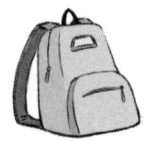

If certain obsessions or compulsions only happen a few times per day but last a long time (like long morning showers), then keep track of how long you spend doing these behaviors or having these thoughts.

Good work today! Next session we're going to learn about the most important way to fight against OCD: exposure and response prevention.

(page 8 of 8)

MODULE 1 HANDOUTS AND WORKSHEETS FOR CHILDREN OR YOUTH

Catch the OCD Bully

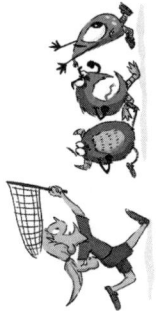

Record the number of times you get stuck on one obsession and one compulsion each day. At the end of the day, write in the totals. Each session we're going to try and get these numbers to shrink! Also, think about how you tried to boss back the OCD and write it down (for example, ignore it, tell it to go away, do something else).

Obsession	Day 1	Day 2	Day 3	Day 4	Day 5	Day 6	Day 7	How I bossed back the OCD bully
	Total:	Total:	Total:	Total:	Total:	Total:	Total:	
Compulsion	Day 1	Day 2	Day 3	Day 4	Day 5	Day 6	Day 7	How I bossed back the OCD bully
	Total:	Total:	Total:	Total:	Total:	Total:	Total:	

From *OCD in Children and Adolescents: The "OCD Is Not the Boss of Me" Manual* by Katherine McKenney, Annie Simpson, and S. Evelyn Stewart. Copyright © 2020 The Guilford Press. Permission to photocopy this material is granted to purchasers of this book for personal use or use with children or youth and their parents (see copyright page for details). Purchasers can download additional copies of this material, in color (see the box at the end of the table of contents).

63

MODULE 1 HANDOUTS AND WORKSHEETS FOR PARENTS

Welcome

Welcome to the treatment program "OCD Is Not the Boss of Me." As parents play an important role in the treatment of pediatric OCD, you will receive handouts over the coming sessions to keep you in touch with how the program works and to even give you some homework of your own to help move your child and family forward on the path to beating OCD. Preferably, these will be given to you at the beginning in advance of your child's session so that you can review their contents and perhaps do some "homework" while your child is with their clinician.

OCD can be a very tricky problem, and you and your child have made the first big step toward letting OCD know that it is "not the boss" in your family. It may well have been a very difficult journey here today and yet you have won the first round by starting this treatment path.

Goals

The handouts that you will be receiving are designed to teach you about OCD and, more importantly, what to do about it. These have been created to address the following five goals:

1. To provide support and encouragement to you as your family begins to take back control of your lives from OCD.
2. To teach you the same strategies your child is learning in their treatment so you can support their efforts at home.
3. To help you to identify and withdraw the subtle (and not-so-subtle) ways your child's OCD is being accommodated.
4. To teach you how to be a cheerleader for your child as they try to boss back the OCD.
5. To teach you how to disengage from angry, conflictual OCD-related interactions with your child.

It is important to also think about what **you** want to accomplish as a result of participating in this program. Your child will be asked today to identify their personal goals for participating in treatment. Take a moment and write down what you want to get out of this, how you would like your family life to be different, or what you would like to be able to do by the end of the program.

My personal goals:

_____

_____

_____

_____

(page 1 of 4)

From *OCD in Children and Adolescents: The "OCD Is Not the Boss of Me" Manual* by Katherine McKenney, Annie Simpson, and S. Evelyn Stewart. Copyright © 2020 The Guilford Press. Permission to photocopy this material is granted to purchasers of this book for personal use or use with children or youth and their parents (see copyright page for details). Purchasers can download additional copies of this material, in color (see the box at the end of the table of contents).

In order to have a good understanding of the tools your child will be learning in their sessions, it is recommended that you read and familiarize yourself with the handouts and worksheets for children or youth. The wonderful thing about these is that they explain OCD and the tools to beat it in a way that is understandable and that will allow you and your child to use the same language and work together as a team. Familiarity with the tools that your child is learning will help support your child in the battle against OCD.

If you wish to learn more about OCD, the following website is a good resource for both you and your child from the International OCD Foundation: *www.ocfoundation.org/ocdinkids*. In addition, connecting with other parents of OCD-affected children may be very beneficial. Depending on your location, regional support groups may be available. Online groups are also helpful in connecting with other parents who have successfully lived through what you are experiencing.

The Importance of Parent Input

Your insights into your child's symptoms and the challenges they encounter at home and at school are extremely important in formulating a treatment plan. Your child will be asked to monitor and report back the frequency and severity of their symptoms for the next several weeks. But we know that children and parents often have very different perspectives on OCD symptoms. So it is important that your child's therapist receives weekly updates from you about what you observe. At each session you will be given a handout in addition to a worksheet to be completed and brought in the following session with observations of your child's OCD behaviors.

Parents' Role in Their Child's OCD Treatment

Parents are often unsure about how active a role they should play in their child's treatment. And this uncertainty may be further complicated by the child's age and maturity level. Ultimately, it is important that children take responsibility for themselves and their treatment. Your job as a parent is to be their **cheerleader**. Acknowledge when they are struggling, praise their efforts, recognize the progress that they've made, and show them that you are confident they can beat the OCD.

You are doing your part as a parent by bringing your child, reading the module handouts, giving feedback on what is happening at home between sessions, and learning how to support your child's efforts.

It can be difficult for parents to take a step back and allow their child to take responsibility for treatment. Here are a few things to remember:

- Parents cannot do the ERPs for their child. They can, however, offer support, encouragement, and rewards for their child's efforts to complete ERPs
- Taking a step back is not the same as punishing your child or abandoning them to face the OCD on their own.
- In fact, allowing your child to take responsibility for their treatment plan is a way of demonstrating your confidence in their ability.
- Given that OCD has the potential to be a lifelong disorder, it is vital that your child learn how to manage the disorder independently.

(page 2 of 4)

The degree to which your child is able to take responsibility for their treatment will vary depending on their age and maturity. Younger children may need (and welcome) daily reminders and assistance to complete ERPs; however, teens may view these same reminders as intrusive and may come to resent your involvement.

A word about homework completion . . . for most families, having a child with OCD causes significant strain and conflict within the home. We don't want to add to that conflict by assigning the role of "homework police" to parents, forcing them to oversee and monitor ERP completion. If your child is having difficulties completing the out-of-session assigned tasks, please let your child's therapist know and they will address it in session. Parents can help by removing any obstacles that may interfere with ERP completion (for example, lack of time, required ERP objects that are not available); however, if the child chooses not to complete the tasks, please allow your child's therapist to deal with this issue directly, rather than becoming a mediator.

Review of Material Covered in the Module 1 Handouts and Worksheets for Children or Youth

The emphasis in Module 1 is on understanding more about OCD. This includes understanding the difference between obsessions and compulsions, and learning about the prevalence of the disorder and the various treatment options (that is, CBT and medication). We introduce the idea of OCD as a "bully in the brain" that the children can boss back. In our program, the OCD bully is represented by the following characters in the materials for children or youth:

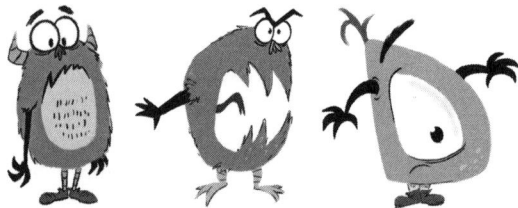

The following concepts and strategies are presented:

Backpacks: Every time a new strategy is discussed in a module, it is identified in the children's manual by a green backpack. This represents the idea that we are teaching the children a number of different strategies that they can use in different situations to manage the OCD.

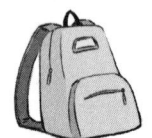

Thought bubbles: The modules are filled with thought bubbles that include "secrets OCD does not want you to know." Once you know the secrets, you are better equipped to boss back the OCD bully. These include facts about OCD and new ways to think differently about the disorder.

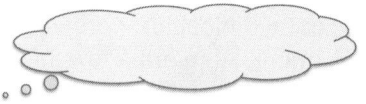

OCD Ruler: This is the first strategy children will be putting in their backpack. Throughout the program, your child will be asked to rate their anxiety, distress, or discomfort on a rating scale from 0 to 10. This allows your child to observe changes in their distress level not only during ERPs (more on that later) but also over the course of the treatment program.

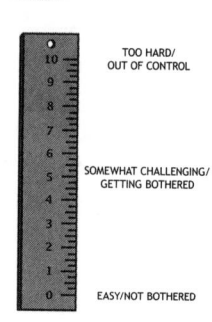

(page 3 of 4)

Catch the OCD bully: This second strategy is designed to not only build greater awareness of OCD symptoms, but to provide a baseline for the severity of your child's symptoms and allow us to record changes over time. Catching the OCD bully involves tracking the frequency of one obsession and one compulsion each day over the course of a week. Your child will be asked to record how often they experience a symptom (or how long it lasts), which will give us a sense of the average frequency of the symptom. Each week your child's therapist will set goals and provide strategies to help lower this number.

Other concepts covered in the children's handouts and worksheets include:

- Setting personal goals for the treatment program.
- Externalizing the OCD so the child begins to see the OCD as something they have, not who they are.
- Understanding the difference between obsessions and compulsions.
- Identifying their own symptoms and deciding what they want to work on first.

MODULE 1 HANDOUTS AND WORKSHEETS FOR PARENTS

Parent Monitoring for Module 1

Each week, monitor the OCD behaviors you observe. These include specific rituals (for example, handwashing, checking), things your child avoids doing, and any OCD-related accommodations that your child requires. Estimate how often these behaviors occur per day and record your response to them (that is, your emotional and/or behavioral reaction). Please bring this sheet with you to the next session.

OCD behaviors (compulsions/ avoidance/demands)	Estimated daily average	Parental response

From OCD in Children and Adolescents: The "OCD Is Not the Boss of Me" Manual by Katherine McKenney, Annie Simpson, and S. Evelyn Stewart. Copyright © 2020 The Guilford Press. Permission to photocopy this material is granted to purchasers of this book for personal use or use with children or youth and their parents (see copyright page for details). Purchasers can download additional copies of this material, in color (see the box at the end of the table of contents).

MODULE 1 HANDOUTS AND WORKSHEETS FOR PARENTS

Therapist Update for Module 1 (to bring to the next session)

Describe any new symptoms that you noticed over the past week:

_____
_____
_____
_____
_____

Describe any particularly challenging OCD situations that occurred over the week:

_____
_____
_____
_____
_____

Describe any successes that your child experienced over the week:

_____
_____
_____
_____
_____

Is there anything else that you think your child's therapist needs to know about the past week? If so, please describe:

_____
_____
_____
_____
_____

From OCD in Children and Adolescents: The "OCD Is Not the Boss of Me" Manual by Katherine McKenney, Annie Simpson, and S. Evelyn Stewart. Copyright © 2020 The Guilford Press. Permission to photocopy this material is granted to purchasers of this book for personal use or use with children or youth and their parents (see copyright page for details). Purchasers can download additional copies of this material, in color (see the box at the end of the table of contents).

MODULE 2

Explaining ERPs, Building an OCD Ladder, and Implementing Rewards

Explaining ERPs to Families

In the previous module, you introduced the concept of ERPs to the parents and their child. Now you have an opportunity to explain in more detail how ERPs work and how to design effective ERPs. Remind the child that the "E" in ERP stands for *exposure*, which involves having them face the trigger, situation, object, image, thought, or idea that typically makes them feel uncomfortable (e.g., anxious, disgusted, "not right"). The "RP" stands for *response prevention*, which is when they ride out the urge to do a compulsion or ritual to neutralize the uncomfortable emotion.

Of course, the above is easier said than done! The majority of individuals with OCD have already attempted to resist compulsions when triggered. If it were so easy to accomplish this, they would not have OCD. This is where the therapist comes in!

Unlike exposures encountered in everyday life, those in ERPs are planned, graduated, and are repeated over and over until they no longer trigger a dysfunctional response of distress-triggered rituals. In fact, when a child or youth complains that the ERPs are getting boring, it's a great sign! It is impossible to be bored and scared at the same time. As well, ERPs *must* be done for an extended period of time. If the child or youth is allowed to escape the exposure by doing compulsions before their anxiety decreases then it actually makes the OCD bully stronger. Remember, avoidance is one of the fuels for anxiety, so we want to make sure that the child experiences success instead of resorting to avoidance!

It is helpful to explain to kids and parents that ERP works in part because of a process of "habituation." The following analogies are helpful to explain this process of habituation that occurs with exposure to distressing situations:

Example 1

"Have you ever tried to jump off the high diving board at the pool or gone on a roller coaster at the amusement park? How did you feel the first time you did it?

"Like most people, you probably felt scared, terrified, and nervous. You may have even tried to back out of it.

"Now imagine you jumped off that diving board or you went on the roller coaster 100 times in a row. How would you feel then?

"The more you do it, the easier it gets. Exposure and response prevention (ERP) activities work the same way. The more you practice, the easier it gets. You get used to it!"

Example 2

"Have you ever seen a horror movie? How did you feel the first time you watched it?

"Now imagine watching that movie 100 times. Pretty boring—huh?

"Why? Because now you know all the scenes by heart, for example, this is the part when the scary monster picks up the knife and chases the girl. Yawn, pretty boring when you know what's going to happen."

It is then helpful to explain the second component of ERP, which is response prevention. This may be done in a manner similar to the following:

"Response prevention involves fighting the urge to do compulsions after you deliberately put yourself in situations that trigger your OCD. When you do ERPs, you are challenging the OCD bully and proving that he is a liar. You'll realize that you can cope with whatever happens. Most importantly, you are taking some of the power away from the OCD bully and giving it back to yourself."

This book details strategies for helping children, youth, and families to fight back against the OCD bully through exposures while changing the compulsion or ritual in a gradual way, enabling further success.

Constructing OCD Ladders

Before starting exposures, it is important to know the situations or behaviors that function as external triggers to obsessions and related compulsions (or avoidance). For example, contamination obsessions (e.g., fears of getting sick) may be triggered by shaking hands with someone, holding the pole on the bus, using the restroom at school, or by having a negative "unacceptable" thought in a specific location. These triggers will produce differing levels of distress, and the child or youth will engage in various physical or mental actions (compulsions) in an effort to neutralize these fears and reduce distress. These actions could include rituals, such as handwashing, spitting, or mental compulsions, as well as avoidance or safety behaviors to ensure that contamination fears do not get triggered in the future (e.g., wearing gloves on the bus, avoiding the use of the bathroom at school, fist bumping to avoid contact with others' palms).

Children and adolescents with OCD almost always have multiple OCD symptom types at once (as described in Chapter 1), each with its own trigger. So how does a therapist know where to begin? The construction of a hierarchy will provide a general road map of where to start and where you're going in treatment with an individual. A fear/aversion hierarchy, termed an *OCD Ladder*, is a list of specific situations or difficulties that trigger OCD-related distress in children or youth. The term *ladder* is helpful in conveying that one starts at the bottom and works their way up, one step at a time. In other words, it conveys that treatment will progress in a controlled and stepwise fashion, building upon small successes to achieve the final goal of bossing back all aspects of OCD.

The construction of an OCD Ladder begins with the child or youth identifying the symptom category that they first want to address. For example, a given individual may report experiencing contamination obsessions, sexual obsessions, and scrupulosity. Rather than tackling all concerns simultaneously, it often works best to select one category of symptoms and build a related OCD Ladder. It should also be explained that there will be opportunities to construct additional ladders for other symptom types as treatment progresses.

Developing an OCD Ladder is a therapeutic process in and of itself, as it allows children and youth to gain an understanding that a distress-provoking trigger can be broken down into manageable components. This realization can subsequently generalize to other OCD symptom categories.

Once the target theme or symptom category has been selected, a brainstorming process can begin. Ask the child or youth to identify situations in which they experience difficulty as a result of OCD, particularly if they are at times unable to resist engaging in a ritual or unable to avoid the situation altogether. For each situation, the child or youth is asked to describe what they think they would do differently if they did not have OCD. For example, if a child or youth's OCD prevents them from entering the kitchen when a parent is preparing food including raw meat, then they could write that if they didn't have OCD, they could: "Stand close to an open package of hamburger." While there are many ways to do this, it helps to write situations on small slips of paper or sticky notes. Of note, it is generally best to identify 10–15 situations, with a minimum of 6–8 situations for a specific OCD Ladder.

CASE EXAMPLE

Simon is a 15-year-old boy who has struggled with OCD for the past 5 years. His symptoms have shifted over time and he is currently struggling with religious obsessions and related avoidance behaviors, praying rituals, and reassurance seeking with parents.

> THERAPIST: Simon, before we can start pushing back against OCD, we need to know where to start. I'd like us to brainstorm a list of situations or activities that are hard for you when you don't do what OCD wants.

SIMON: What do you mean? I don't get it. Everything is hard because of OCD.

THERAPIST: It sounds like OCD is really overwhelming for you right now. I'm talking about things that would make you feel really anxious unless you do an OCD ritual. You told me earlier that it's hard for you to drive past churches and that OCD makes you repeat a prayer in your head over and over again when you do.

SIMON: Yeah, sometimes I'll still be saying the prayer 20 minutes after I get home.

THERAPIST: So, driving past churches is something that is hard for you right now. Let's write that down on this small slip of paper. What other things are hard related to the thought that comes into your head about displeasing God?

Together, Simon and his therapist developed the following list of potential rungs on his OCD Ladder:

- Driving past a church
- Watching Harry Potter or other movies about witchcraft or the occult
- Writing the number "6"
- Reading about other religions
- Talking to people from other religions
- Saying grace before meals
- Hearing others curse
- Saying curse words
- Listening to music with offensive lyrics
- Walking in areas where insects (God's creatures) could be stepped on

Once 10–15 situations have been generated, the child or youth should be asked to estimate their expected level of distress if they were to encounter each situation at present. They will then write the distress score (i.e., SUDs/the OCD Ruler number) on the slip of paper. These distress ratings should be based on predictions of how the child or youth would feel if they were faced with that situation and they did not carry out a related ritual or avoidance behavior.

After the situations have been rated, the child or youth should be asked to arrange them on the OCD Ladder worksheet with the least distressing situation at the bottom and the most distressing situation at the top. Of note, it is not necessary to identify situations that represent each numerical point on the scale. It is fine to have multiple situations rated as a 5, for example, as long as there is some distribution throughout the whole scale across identified situations.

It is important that the child identify a range of distress-provoking situations on their OCD Ladder so that they can begin with ERPs in low-distress-provoking situations before proceeding to moderate- and high-distress-provoking situations. Beginning with a relatively easy situation will enable the child or youth to firmly establish their ERP skills and ensure early experiences of success and confidence. This will optimize motivation and willingness to tackle more difficult situations later in therapy. In the path to beating OCD, success breeds success.

Returning to Simon, based on his ratings, he and his therapist developed the following OCD Ladder for his scrupulosity fears:

	OCD Ruler rating (0–10)
Saying curse words	10
Watching Harry Potter or other movies about witchcraft or the occult	9
Writing the number "6"	9
Driving past a church	8
Saying grace before meals	8
Talking to people from other religions	6
Hearing others curse	5
Listening to music with offensive lyrics	5
Walking in areas where insects (God's creatures) could be stepped on	4
Reading about other religions	3

THERAPIST: Simon, you've done a great job at building your OCD Ladder. We've got a nice balance of ideas for situations that are at the bottom, middle, and top of your ladder.

SIMON: Yeah, but there's no way you're going to get me to say any curse words.

THERAPIST: I know that the top of your ladder feels like an impossible challenge right now. That's why we don't start at the top. We'll start with steps that are challenging but not overwhelming and gradually work our way up. And remember, each step on the ladder can be broken down into small challenges.

SIMON: I get it, but I'm still not gonna swear.

THERAPIST: I hear you, Simon. Right now, swearing is not something you're willing to do yet. Let's see how you feel about it in a few weeks after you've been working on ERPs for a bit.

The OCD Ladder is a road map that will guide which exposures are attempted and in what order. It provides direction to inform treatment planning, rather than a rigid rule set that requires strict adherence. The OCD Ladder ratings will change as children and youth habituate to various triggers. What had previously been defined as an "8" may soon become only a "4." Some situations may no longer be triggering, even though they have not been specifically used as exposures. This is because habituation in one situation may generalize to other situations. When a specific OCD domain has been conquered, treatment should shift to other symptom categories, for which new OCD Ladders can be created. Each ladder will be broken down into specific ERP tasks to be attempted.

Potential OCD Ladder Pitfalls

Sometimes OCD symptoms can themselves interfere with constructing an OCD Ladder. Here are some common situations and ways to address them:

- Children or youth with perfectionistic tendencies may perseverate on identifying the most accurate SUDs rating or on developing the "best" triggering exposure situation. In these cases, allowing them to remain stuck and to ruminate about the best response is actually reinforcing OCD symptoms. These individuals may benefit from ignoring specific SUDs ratings and by focusing on whether tasks will be "easy," "moderate," or "difficult" to accomplish. They may also benefit from knowing that OCD Ladders are not "written in stone," rather that they are meant to be fluid and flexible and are expected to change over time.

- Children or youth with erasing and rewriting symptoms may find the act of writing out triggering situations to be triggering in and of itself. For these individuals, the therapist can act as a scribe. In case you are wondering as you read this, "But isn't this accommodation?" you are correct. However, as always the risks and benefits of any action must be weighed against each other. In this case, accommodation is facilitating a necessary step in planning treatment. The accommodation should be noted to the child or youth and parents, with the encouraging message that they should be able to write on their own, without help, by the time they complete their journey in bossing back OCD.

Establishing a Reward System

The reward program should be considered an integral component of OCD ERP treatment, not an afterthought. One reason why children and youth may fail to make gains in treatment is because reward programs have been implemented inconsistently or the rewards themselves are not meaningful for the individual. Setting aside time in session to outline a comprehensive reward program is essential to reaping payoff later in treatment.

ERPs are hard work and are, by definition, always aversive since no one wants to deliberately make themselves feel anxious, uncomfortable, or distraught. Prior to treatment, efforts at resisting OCD will have generally only resulted in negative feelings. By rewarding an individual attempting ERPs, the previously held association begins to change, such that resisting OCD becomes paired with a positive outcome—the reward! Rewards also can instill motivation to take on the difficult work of ERPs in those who are otherwise ambivalent. Hence, it is very important for both therapists and parents to have a reward program in place before actively engaging in treatment. When working together to build an effective reward system, here are some points to keep in mind:

Timing of Rewards

Rewards must follow rather than precede completion of ERP assignments. Although this probably seems obvious to most therapists, it is important to ensure that parents and the child understand that as well. Not infrequently, a parent may give their child a video game, privilege, or other item that they can "pay off" with future ERPs. However, once received, the reward loses its motivating influence for their child and opens the door to procrastination. In addition, this may set up a challenging precedent in which the child or youth demands increasing rewards, which become associated with false promises and debating skills, rather than actual attempts to "face the OCD bully."

A reward is most effective when received soon after challenge completion. This allows it to be most tightly paired with the self-pride and surprised disbelief experienced after a child or youth has faced a challenge previously thought to be impossible. A reward that a child must wait all week to receive will very quickly lose its appeal, particularly when the disincentive of needing to complete further ERP exercises is high and immediate.

Appropriate Targets for Rewards

Rewards should be earned for attempting or completing a task, rather than for a perfect performance. They are also not earned by reports of decreasing distress, as this can inadvertently encourage false reports of symptom improvement.

If a child or youth does not attempt an assigned ERP task, they should not be provided with a reward. It is very important, although sometimes difficult, for both therapists and parents to apply this consistently. Children or youth with recent or past experiences of earning rewards following ERP may begin to "check the limits" of what is required to continue receiving them. Given therapist and parent investment in the child's gains and engagement in the treatment process, it may be particularly difficult to withhold a planned reward or to resist "renegotiating" expectations and requirements for the reward.

When a child or youth refuses to attempt previously agreed-upon ERP homework, it may also be tempting for parents to give their child extra attention. This may involve engagement in long, drawn-out discussions, focusing on how distressed the child may become, potential downsides to attempting homework, "fairness" or safety of the homework, uncertainty about the child's ability to withstand the challenge, and so forth. This is unhelpful on many levels:

1. It teaches the child that procrastination is effective in avoiding fears (e.g., as opposed to "just doing it").
2. It provides positive reinforcement via extra parental attention (from the child's perspective, additional parental attention is usually better).

3. It challenges roles that have been established, with the therapist as the ERP homework assigner and the parent as the "cheerleader/supporter."

Rather than rewarding a child for not attempting ERP homework, as described above, parents should be encouraged to report back at the next session (without judgment), such that future ERP assignments will have greater chances of success.

How to Reward

Families are more likely to stick with a reward program if they use charts or written documentation for tracking OCD homework and associated rewards. This also helps to provide clarity and minimize debates between sessions regarding expectations.

What to Provide as a Reward

Behavioral rewards can take many forms, and the age of the child or youth will determine the nature of the reward. A reward system is more effective when a therapist can work with children, youth, and parents collaboratively to develop a list. This allows the child or youth to identify what is motivating to them and to increase their ownership and "buy-in" to the system. It also ensures that parents agree about the rewards and are able to provide them consistently as planned.

Rewards must be something special and not otherwise easily available to the child or youth. Rewards are not effective as motivators if the child will receive it whether or not they engage in ERP (e.g., having a youth "earn" a winter coat, when all children in the family get a new coat each year). Rewards should generally be small and relatively inexpensive. For children and youth who are most motivated by a specific bigger reward, tokens can be earned toward acquiring this. However, the related aspect of delayed gratification may limit effectiveness and perceived reinforcement of this approach.

Rewards should be proportional to the level of OCD challenge being faced. In other words, agree upon little rewards for small challenges and bigger rewards for more distress-provoking tasks.

Brainstorming a list of all possible rewards with the child, youth, and parents is a good first step. This should be an open, fun, unrestricted brainstorming session. Ideas that are impractical, unreasonable, or not feasible can subsequently be removed or altered in a more grounded discussion following brainstorming.

Reward Suggestions

Not every reward is going to be motivating for every child or youth. What appeals to an 8-year-old will not necessarily appeal to a 16-year-old. The child or youth is usually the best equipped to know which rewards would make them most inclined to work hard. The chart below offers reward suggestions for different age groups.

Age	Reward
Young children	Stickers, gum, bubbles, Hershey kisses/gummy bears/small candies, temporary tattoos, privileges, special time with parents, access to reserved toys (e.g., electronic gaming systems)
Elementary school	Special activities (e.g., local pool, climbing gym), toys, screen time, time alone with parents and without siblings
Preteen	Screen time, access to desired activities, apps, gift cards, $$$, privileges
High school	Gas cards, gift cards, access to the car, apps, texting time, later curfew, $$$, privileges

If the child selects a large reward and plans to earn credits or points toward its purchase, here are some creative ways to provide more immediate and tangible reinforcement of ERP attempts along the way:

- Have parents purchase a desired video game, and then children earn time to play that game instead of earning money toward making the purchase at a later date.
- Earn components that can be used with the larger reward. For example, if the child will be getting a hamster at the end of treatment, then they can earn the cage, the wheel, and the food along the way.
- Print off a large image of the desired item and cut it into puzzle pieces. With each completed ERP, the child earns a piece of the puzzle. Once the puzzle is complete, they receive the larger reward.

What *Not* to Provide as a Reward

Rewards should be entirely independent of OCD-related core fears, avoidance, or ritualistic behavior. If not, ERP gains by the child or youth will result in rewards that actually reinforce and negatively impact their illness. We include this paragraph as related situations may not be overtly obvious. As with other aspects of OCD treatment, reward decisions should be highly individualized based upon illness presentation. Consider the example of Internet access time as a reward. While this is a strong and appropriate reward motivator for many, it should not be used for children and youth who rely upon the Internet for rituals such as checking weather reports, disease characteristics, emergent disaster stories, and so on. Other examples of unadvisable rewards in related specific circumstances include cleaning products or replacement clothing/items (with contamination obsessions), extra visits to synagogue/church (with religious obsessions), later bedtimes (with redoing of homework), and drives to school (with OCD-related bus avoidance).

Addressing Parental Concerns about Rewards

The following questions are frequently raised when discussing rewards with parents.

"Isn't This Bribing My Child to Work on Their OCD?"

No, a reward system is about acknowledging the effort the child has made to address the OCD so that they will be more motivated to do the same again in the future. Remember, a reward comes after the behavior, whereas a bribe comes before. Also, a bribe is tied to some additional benefit for the individual providing it, whereas a reward is simply intended to benefit the recipient. Last, bribes are typically provided to encourage unethical behavior, which is not the case for rewards.

"Shouldn't My Child Have Enough Motivation to Do ERPs without Rewards?"

The treatment for OCD requires a lot of hard work that is often uncomfortable, even initially terrifying for children and youth. It is unrealistic to expect them to embrace the treatment with open arms. A reward system can move the treatment process along by providing additional motivators to encourage them to do homework, practice ERPs, and so forth. Remember, not many adults would show up to work if they weren't being paid—isn't a salary one of the biggest reward systems of all?

Parents may also wonder why their child would choose to live with OCD, suggesting that, if they were truly suffering, their OCD improvement should be reward enough in itself. However, this ignores potential worries by their child that things will worsen, in addition to a fear of the unknown. In this situation, children may strongly identify with the expression "Better the devil you know than the devil you don't."

"Isn't This Going to Be Really Expensive?"

Rewards do not need to be costly. Rewards may include "special time" between a parent and a child or a special privilege such as choosing what food will be prepared for dinner. Parents can consider placing a greater emphasis on privileges rather than on material items, such as offering a later bedtime, extra screen time, or double dessert. No matter the type of reward, remind parents that any reward system is going to be cheaper than a lifetime of managing their child's untreated OCD.

"Am I Going to Have to Reward My Child Forever?"

No. In fact, a good reward system also has a plan for discontinuation, because it is the effort rather than the specific behavior that is being reinforced. Over time, as the child or youth completes sequential ERP homework, they are enabled to take on greater challenges. And previous challenges require less effort and cause less distress, thereby earning smaller, and eventually no, rewards. For example, if the child or youth initially earned an extra 30 minutes of screen time for doing one ERP, they will soon be required to complete two ERPs in order to earn that same additional screen time. With each success, the child's internal motivation also tends to grow, making external rewards less relevant. However, praise and encouragement from parents and therapists is always required!

"What If My Child Isn't Motivated by Rewards?"

It is rare for a child or youth to be unmotivated by any possible reward. When this strategy is not working for a family, it may be that the particular rewards being used are not motivating, are being delivered after too long a delay, or that the work being asked of the child or youth is too aversive to them. Sometimes families need to be creative and think "outside the box" to generate reward ideas.

Some children and youth with scrupulosity OCD symptoms (i.e., marked concern with morality, fairness, and selflessness) may initially refuse all rewards. One approach in such cases is to contribute a certain amount toward a charity of their choice for attempting an ERP challenge. While this admittedly contradicts the advice above to not offer rewards related to OCD symptoms, flexibility may be required to enable success! Later ERPs for these children and youth may actually include tolerating the distress of accepting rewards for themselves.

Sample Dialogue (Early Conversation)

THERAPIST: Jilly, you are going to be working very hard, and so today we are going to come up with some prizes to reward you for all your hard work! What kinds of things do you think you might like?

JILLY: Oh no, I don't need rewards, I'll just do it. I don't really like prizes. Anyway, my little sister will be so jealous. Plus, I really don't want my parents wasting their money on me—especially when there are starving kids in the world.

THERAPIST: Well, it is really important that we pick something . . . so what do you like?

JILLY: Really—nothing . . . I promise I'll work hard.

THERAPIST: So I heard you mention starving kids. Is that something you really care about?

JILLY: Well, of course it is! Doesn't everyone?

THERAPIST: So, what if your prize for hard work is money for you to donate to a charity that you pick?

JILLY: Well, I guess that would be okay.

As treatment progressed, Jilly began to earn money toward an activity that she and her sister could do together. At the end of treatment, Jilly was able to name a prize that she herself wanted, and started saving toward that.

In some families, children and youth have free and complete access to computers, TV, cell phones, toys, and so forth. In other words, it can be hard to identify extra privileges for those who already have access to everything. In those cases, it may be necessary for families to implement some limits so that there is something to work toward.

Children will sometimes request (and receive) rewards that are inappropriately extravagant and cannot be sustained over time. Sometimes parents offer more than they can afford in the hopes of gaining faster improvements in treatment. The following case example illustrates how a therapist might navigate these situations.

CASE EXAMPLE

John is a 9-year-old boy who has significant contamination obsessions related to fears of getting sick, which he neutralizes through excessive handwashing, extended showers, and the use of barriers. His parents have been accommodating the OCD by providing extra soap, doing extra laundry, and remaining with John in the bathroom while he showers (as requested) to minimize his distress. They are exhausted and desperate for things to improve at home.

> THERAPIST: Welcome back, everyone. After our session last week, I sent you off with a homework task to make a list of possible rewards for attempted ERPs. What did you come up with?
>
> JOHN: I really want to go to Disneyland, and Mom and Dad said we could go if I get over my OCD.
>
> THERAPIST: Wow! Disneyland would be a lot of fun. We might need to think about how to break down that big reward into smaller rewards that you can earn for daily ERP practice. If you were to go to Disneyland, would you want to buy some souvenirs when you're there?
>
> JOHN: Oh yeah. I'd want to get mouse ears, and a T-shirt, and a toy, and a stuffie, and . . .
>
> THERAPIST: That sounds awesome. So, earning a small amount of money that you could put toward buying souvenirs would be a good thing that you would want. Mom and Dad, what do you think about that idea?
>
> MOM: That would be fine. John could earn $10 for every ERP he tries.
>
> THERAPIST: That's a lot of money, especially since we want John to practice multiple ERPs several times each day.
>
> DAD: That's way too much money. One dollar seems more reasonable.
>
> THERAPIST: I agree. So, for every time John attempts an ERP, he can earn $1 to spend at Disneyland. John, are there any special things you want to do at Disneyland?
>
> JOHN: I want to get photos with my favorite characters.
>
> THERAPIST: I like to do that at Disneyland too. So maybe you could earn a photo when you try some of the really challenging ERPs at the top of your fear ladder?
>
> JOHN: Okay. And I can keep track of how many photos I've earned.
>
> THERAPIST: Sounds great. Mom and Dad, do you agree with that plan? We want to make sure we're coming up with rewards for when John tries ERPs, not for him totally getting over OCD. This is because trying the ERPs is the thing that will lead to his improvement.

What about the Idea of Punishing the Child or Youth to Stop the OCD Behaviors?

Parents often consider implementing punishments to address OCD symptoms (e.g., punishing their child for engaging in rituals). Unfortunately, punishments typically serve to drive the rituals out of the parents' view rather than making them go away, since their child tries to prevent them from detecting compulsions to avoid being punished. This tends to increase the degree of secrecy surrounding OCD and interferes with effective treatment planning, as parents may perceive the symptoms to be less severe or impairing given that they are not easily observable. Children and youth are then left to suffer with the disorder on their own in isolation.

How Far to Go in Exposures?

A commonly addressed question by novice OCD therapists, as well as by seasoned clinicians, is that of "how far to go" when conducting exposures. Specific questions include: Is there such a thing as too far? Why do we ask kids to do things that those without OCD would never do?

Experienced OCD therapists may proudly describe the most extreme exposures they have done with children or youth (and the positive impact it had on their symptoms!). We have personally (or know therapists who have) done the following in the course of an ERP: jumped into dumpsters, eaten candy from toilet seats, held raw chicken then eaten candy afterwards, had children hold knives to their throats, smoked a cigarette in close proximity to the child or youth's face, licked the bathroom floor, and voiced obscenities in public. The potential list of "extreme" exposures is endless. From the outside, this may appear to be driven by a sadistic or competitive drive to create the most disgusting, morally or otherwise reprehensible challenge. However, therapists familiar with OCD-specific ERP are aware that these are not the goals, and that ERPs are guided by specific, core OCD fears of the individual child or youth.

It could be asked why therapists challenge the child or youth to do these things. In order to be effective, ERPs must target core fears and prevent the avoidance or rituals associated with them. It is important to leave "no stone unturned" in the course of therapy, such that all OCD symptom areas are addressed, thereby minimizing the risk for relapse. The importance of "overcorrection," or doing things that people without OCD typically would not do should be explained.

There are several reasons why overcorrection in ERPs is important:

1. Life is unpredictable and the goal is to build the child or youth's confidence to cope with any daily circumstance.
2. To ensure remission, it is important that the child does not minimize their gains by telling themselves that "the bad thing didn't happen because I didn't actually come fully in contact with the real danger." This reassurance safety ritual would thus interfere with gaining generalization. It is therefore important to address items

at the very top of the child or youth's hierarchy, and even beyond, such that OCD's threatening messages have been addressed.

It can at times be difficult to get "buy-in" and convince a child or youth (and their parents) to engage in these more challenging exposures. It can be helpful to have a conversation comparing what life looks like now and in the future with OCD, versus the risk of what they are being asked to do. For example, compared to a life spent in one's basement hiding from OCD, the (realistically low) risk of eating a jellybean rubbed on a toilet seat is a small price to pay! Similarly, a discussion about what their lives look like with OCD, and what they will be able to do once OCD "takes a hike" can also increase motivation. (e.g., "I'll have more time with my friends"; "I'll be on time for school"; "I'll be able to go to sleepovers").

As an OCD therapist, it is critical to motivate, encourage, and supportively push OCD-affected children and youth to do exposures that deliberately make them feel distressed. The experience of tolerating these uncomfortable feelings without ritualizing is critical for the individual to eventually beat OCD. This concept may sometimes go against the natural instincts of therapists, who are drawn to the field with a goal of making others feel better by relieving suffering. The worry that exposures may potentially cause harmful "trauma" can also trouble therapists. Confusion may arise from the misguided notion that uncomfortable feelings are bad in and of themselves. However, negative and uncomfortable feelings are an inherent part of life. Bad feelings come and go on their own and doing rituals to manage or avoid these will only lead to entrenchment of OCD. Helping children and youth learn how to manage discomfort is a skill that cannot be overvalued.

When a child exhibits oppositional behavior, reluctance, and fear about completing a planned exposure, it may be tempting for a therapist to pull back. However, it is precisely at these times, that therapists must persevere as much as possible. Ignoring these behaviors (e.g., crying, whining, protesting, screaming) and being firm but supportive will help children or youth to push through uncomfortable feelings. Supportive statements can go a long way in increasing motivation and willingness. Examples of these include: "I know you can do this," "You are a rock star OCD fighter," and "Remember the time you did X exposure and sent OCD running in fear?" The therapist's job is to push! Sometimes this can require building one's own tolerance of negative emotions as therapists. It can be troubling to seemingly contribute to a child or youth's distress. But keeping focused on the final goal can help therapists to tolerate the child's short-term negative feelings.

When the Child or Youth Refuses an Exposure

If, despite encouragement and persistence, a child continues to refuse to attempt an exposure, never allow full avoidance. Instead, go back to the last situation in which the child was successful and attempt that again. It is generally a good approach for the therapist to take ownership of the failed exposure with a statement such as the following: "Okay, I messed up with that exposure—it's my fault for making one too hard too soon, Let's go back to X, which you really rocked, and next time we will go slower." It is important to highlight the fact that you will continue to work together toward whatever exposure was initially planned, and to express confidence that eventually they will be able to successfully tackle it.

So, how far is too far? Pushing too far too fast runs the risk of losing the child or youth's engagement in therapy and a refusal to continue with crucial ERPs. Furthermore, therapists must always be careful to avoid harm due to the treatment itself. See Module 7 if the child refuses to do any exposures at all.

Ensuring Engagement

Several principles can help guide therapists to ensure engagement in best practices:

1. Follow the rule of thumb articulated in the following question: "Does this exposure put myself or the child or youth at significantly greater risk than we would typically encounter in our daily lives?"
2. Always conduct a proper and thorough assessment to ensure that exposure exercises are targeting a core OCD fear.
3. Ensure ERPs are relevant and of interest to the child or youth, which often means finding a "hook" (e.g., sports, a specific TV show, or a fictional character of interest to the child) that will make the ERP more meaningful. Creatively integrating a child or youth's interests into exposures may help to ensure engagement.
4. Use of humor in therapy is important to remove some of the perceived seriousness from OCD.
5. Treat the child or youth as an active participant in treatment plan development—have them contribute to the design of each exposure. With time, you may find that they are coming up with exposures that even you feel too uncomfortable to perform!
6. If an exposure appears to be too difficult for the child or youth, break it down into smaller manageable steps.
7. Never ask children or youths to do something that you as a therapist are unwilling to do along with them, or that has a reasonable chance of causing significant harm to themselves, someone else, or property.
8. Consult with others on a regular basis to ensure that you are choosing appropriate exposures. This should not be limited to consultation with colleagues and supervisors, but should involve authorities in different areas as needed. For example, consult with religious figures (e.g., priests, rabbis) when doing exposures around scrupulosity to ensure that you are not asking people to do exposures that go against religious beliefs as typically practiced in their faith community.

Homework Assignments

For Module 2, therapists can assign the following for youth and parents to complete at home before the next session:

For Youth
- Complete the Catch the OCD Bully worksheet (symptom monitoring).

- Practice at least one ERP daily between sessions.
- With parents, brainstorm a list of possible rewards to earn for attempting ERPs.

For Parents

- Complete the Parent Monitoring worksheet (parent observations of various compulsions, avoidance behaviors, and accommodations that the child requires, as well as estimated per-day average of each, and how parents responded).
- Complete the Therapist Update worksheet. This worksheet allows parents to share with the child's therapist any new OCD symptoms that were observed over the week, any particularly challenging OCD situations the family encountered, any successes the child experienced, and any other information parents feel would be helpful for the therapist to know. Therapists should ask parents to provide them with this completed worksheet at the start of the next session so they can address specific issues as needed with the child or with the whole family together.
- With youth, develop a contract that outlines rewards earned for various ERPs.

MODULE 2 HANDOUTS AND WORKSHEETS FOR CHILDREN OR YOUTH

Building Your Ladder

Last session we learned that, just like with schoolyard bullies, you have to stand up to the OCD bully and not go along with what it wants you to do. It's hard to stand up to the OCD bully . . . every person with OCD has tried at some point to not give in to OCD's demands. One way to make it easier is to start being brave and resist OCD in small ways and in easier situations. With practice, you'll be able to stand up to the OCD bully in tougher and tougher situations until you're able to stand up to the bully entirely.

One way to do this is to build an OCD Ladder. An OCD Ladder is a list of situations where the OCD bully causes problems for you. OCD Ladders are organized with easier situations on the bottom, medium situations in the middle, and harder situations near the top. Just like climbing a real ladder, you're going to start at the bottom and work your way up **AT YOUR OWN PACE.**

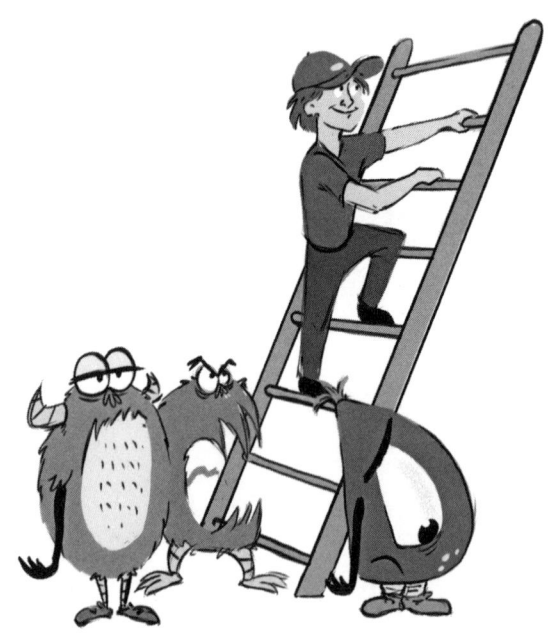

OCD Ladders should be about one type of OCD worry. So if the OCD bully is making you worry about getting sick, doubt that the doors are locked, or feel that things just aren't right, pick one topic and create your OCD ladder around that.

Start by writing down situations where OCD is causing problems for you on slips of paper. Try to think of at least six to eight situations. Then group them into categories based on how difficult it would be for you to get through these situations without doing what OCD wants. You can use the OCD Ruler to score the situations and organize them from easiest to most challenging, or just group them into categories of "easy," "medium," and "hard." Remember, everyone's OCD is unique, so everyone's OCD Ladder is going to be unique!

It's Time to Start Building Your Ladder!

After you've organized the situations into groups, fill in the OCD Ladder on the next page.

(page 1 of 4)

From *OCD in Children and Adolescents: The "OCD Is Not the Boss of Me" Manual* by Katherine McKenney, Annie Simpson, and S. Evelyn Stewart. Copyright © 2020 The Guilford Press. Permission to photocopy this material is granted to purchasers of this book for personal use or use with children or youth and their parents (see copyright page for details). Purchasers can download additional copies of this material, in color (see the box at the end of the table of contents).

OCD Ladder

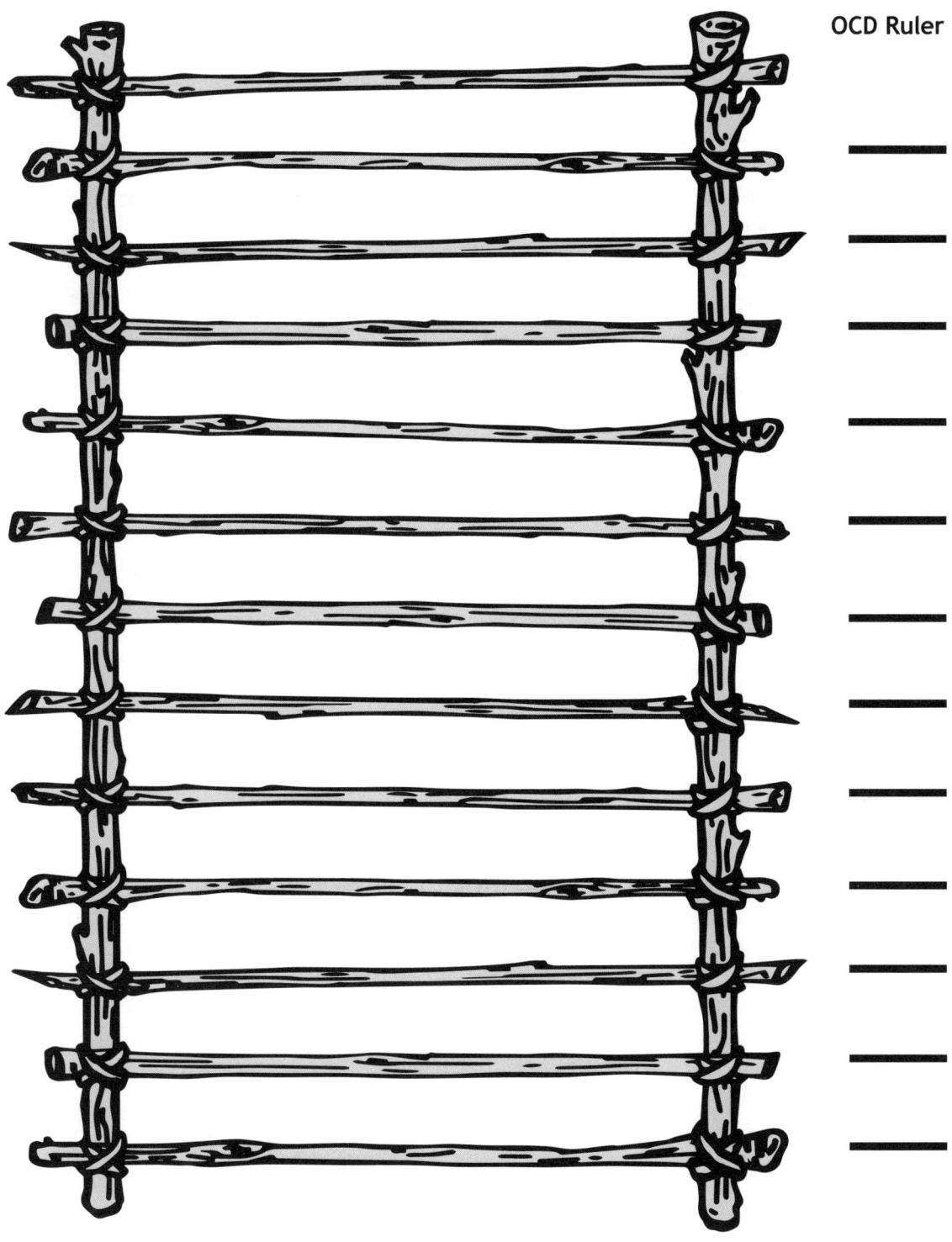

OCD Ruler

(page 2 of 4)

Your OCD Ladder isn't set in stone. You and your therapist will probably make changes to it as you go along. You'll probably also make several OCD Ladders for different symptoms. As you start to climb your ladder, you may think of OCD situations that you want to add, remove, or change. You may also discover that some of the steps are too big to manage. Don't worry if that happens. You can always break steps down into smaller steps. You get to make the decisions about the size of your steps. Remember, your ladder is a work in progress!

Now we're going to use information on your OCD Ladder to start setting some limits on your obsessions and compulsions using exposure and response prevention, or ERP.

Exposure and Response Prevention (ERP)

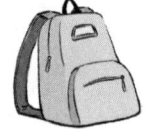

Have you ever tried to jump off the high diving board at the pool?

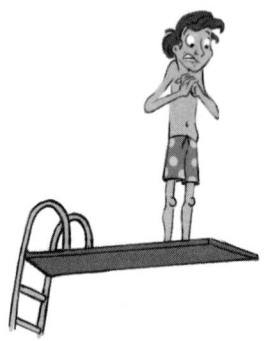

How did you feel the first time you did it? _____

_____.

Like most people, you probably felt scared, terrified, and nervous. You may have even tried to back out of it. Now imagine you jump off that diving board 100 times in a row. How would you feel then?

_____

_____

_____.

The more you do it, the easier it gets. Exposure and response prevention (ERP) activities work the same way. The more you practice, the easier it gets.

ERP is the most effective strategy in your fight to boss back the OCD bully. Exposure (the *E* in ERP) means facing your fears until your uncomfortable feelings go down on their own. This process is called "habituation." It's just like jumping off the high diving board . . . eventually you're no longer scared of doing it because you got used to it.

Response prevention (the *RP* in ERP) involves fighting the urge to do compulsions when you deliberately put yourself in situations that trigger your anxiety or make you feel gross or just "not right." When you do ERPs, you are challenging the OCD bully and proving that he is a liar. You'll realize that you can cope with whatever happens. Most importantly, you are taking some of the power away from the OCD bully and giving it back to yourself.

When doing ERPs there are three things to keep in mind:

1. You need to do each step on your OCD Ladder **over and over** again until it no longer bothers you. Keep doing a step until you're bored with it!

2. You need to do the ERPs **as often as possible**. So you need to practice the same step often and many times. You should plan to practice at least once per day. The more you work at it, the faster you'll get your OCD under control.

3. You need to keep doing the ERP for **a long, extended period of time** to allow your uncomfortable feelings to naturally decrease. If you stop the ERP too soon, the OCD bully may get a little stronger.

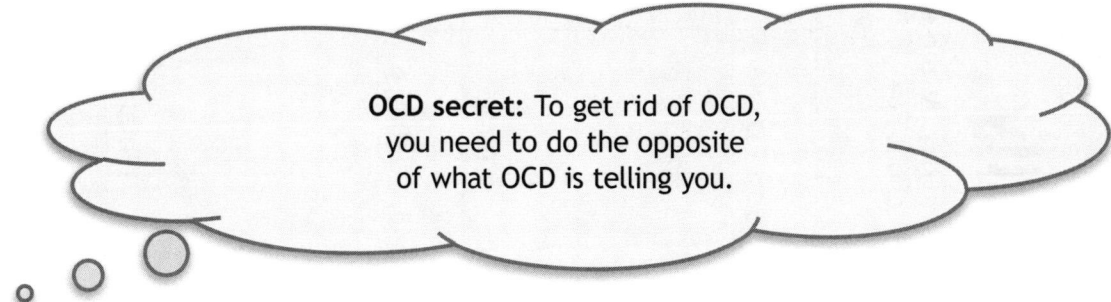

OCD secret: To get rid of OCD, you need to do the opposite of what OCD is telling you.

For homework this week, you are going to start climbing up your OCD Ladder, beginning with the first step! You're going to start with one step at a time and you won't move on to the next step until you've mastered the previous one. We'll use the information on your OCD Ladder to develop your first ERP for homework.

(page 4 of 4)

MODULE 2 HANDOUTS AND WORKSHEETS FOR CHILDREN OR YOUTH

Catch the OCD Bully

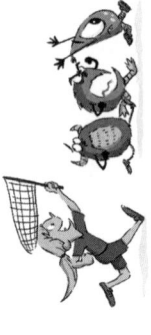

Record the number of times you get stuck on one obsession and one compulsion each day. At the end of the day, write in the totals. Each session we're going to try and get these numbers to shrink! Also, think about how you tried to boss back the OCD and write it down (for example, ignore it, tell it to go away, do something else).

Obsession	Day 1	Day 2	Day 3	Day 4	Day 5	Day 6	Day 7	How I bossed back the OCD bully
	Total:	Total:	Total:	Total:	Total:	Total:	Total:	
Compulsion	Day 1	Day 2	Day 3	Day 4	Day 5	Day 6	Day 7	How I bossed back the OCD bully
	Total:	Total:	Total:	Total:	Total:	Total:	Total:	

From *OCD in Children and Adolescents: The "OCD Is Not the Boss of Me" Manual* by Katherine McKenney, Annie Simpson, and S. Evelyn Stewart. Copyright © 2020 The Guilford Press. Permission to photocopy this material is granted to purchasers of this book for personal use or use with children or youth and their parents (see copyright page for details). Purchasers can download additional copies of this material, in color (see the box at the end of the table of contents).

MODULE 2 HANDOUTS AND WORKSHEETS FOR CHILDREN OR YOUTH

ERP Home Practice for Module 2

What is the OCD bully trying to trick you into believing?	ERP	Goal for the week	Daily ERP results
			Day 1:
			Day 2:
			Day 3:
			Day 4:
			Day 5:
			Day 6:
			Day 7:
			Day 1:
			Day 2:
			Day 3
			Day 4:
			Day 5
			Day 6:
			Day 7:

From *OCD in Children and Adolescents: The "OCD Is Not the Boss of Me" Manual* by Katherine McKenney, Annie Simpson, and S. Evelyn Stewart. Copyright © 2020 The Guilford Press. Permission to photocopy this material is granted to purchasers of this book for personal use or use with children or youth and their parents (see copyright page for details). Purchasers can download additional copies of this material, in color (see the box at the end of the table of contents).

MODULE 2 HANDOUTS AND WORKSHEETS FOR PARENTS

ERPs and Behavioral Rewards

Today you and your child will begin learning about the most important and effective tool for beating back their OCD: exposure and response prevention (ERP). This behavioral technique is the foundation of their treatment program—your child will be asked to complete ERPs both in session and at home between sessions for the remainder of the program. Therefore it is key that you as a parent have a good understanding of this tool and the ways you can support your child with their ERP homework.

In today's module you'll also focus on the importance of developing an effective reward program that will encourage your child to practice their ERPs.

Review of Material Covered in the Module 2 Handouts and Worksheets for Children or Youth

Exposure and Response Prevention (ERP): ERP is the most effective form of behavioral therapy for addressing OCD. ERP involves triggering the child's obsessive fears (exposure) while at the same time supporting and encouraging the child to not engage in those compulsions that are designed to reduce the obsession-related distress (response prevention). With repeated exposures, the child's distress decreases through a process called habituation. The following graph shows how your child's distress rises in response to an obsessive thought and decreases after they engage in a ritual.

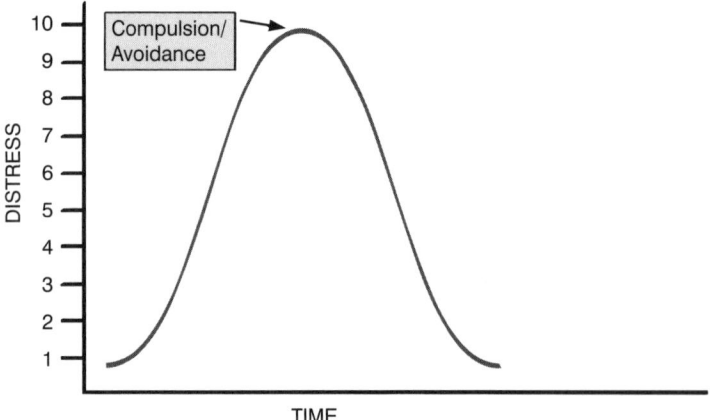

The next graph illustrates what happens if your child is triggered by a thought but resists the urge to do their compulsion. Initially their distress level remains high, but soon it begins to decrease on its own through habituation. With regular and consistent practice, your child will become less distressed by the obsessive thought and will be able to more easily resist compulsions.

(page 1 of 4)

From *OCD in Children and Adolescents: The "OCD Is Not the Boss of Me" Manual* by Katherine McKenney, Annie Simpson, and S. Evelyn Stewart. Copyright © 2020 The Guilford Press. Permission to photocopy this material is granted to purchasers of this book for personal use or use with children or youth and their parents (see copyright page for details). Purchasers can download additional copies of this material, in color (see the box at the end of the table of contents).

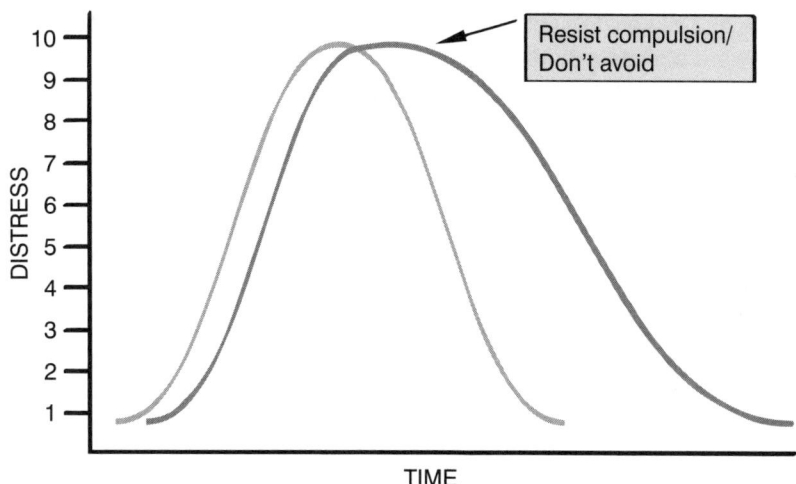

OCD Ladder: An OCD Ladder provides a visual map that represents your child's OCD symptoms and related distress. Together with their therapist, your child will generate a list of situations and activities that will trigger their obsessions and subsequent distress. These situations will be ranked in order from lowest score on the OCD Ruler to the highest. This predetermined list will allow your child to work through ERPs in a graded fashion. In other words, milder symptoms and triggers are attempted first. As treatment progresses, more difficult exposures are presented. By practicing milder, less distressing exposures first, your child is more likely to experience successful habituation, which will lead to a greater willingness to attempt more challenging exposures later on.

Behavioral Rewards (a Key to Success!!!)

ERPs are a lot of hard work and are not particularly enjoyable (no one wants to deliberately make themself feel anxious or uncomfortable). That is why it is really important that families have a reward program in place to help motivate the child to practice their ERPs. Rewards can take many forms and the age of your child will determine the nature of the reward.

Many parents many feel as though their child should have enough internal motivation to deal with the OCD and complete their ERPs without any external incentives. Remember, your child would not be participating in treatment if they did not want to get better. The treatment for OCD is challenging so your child will need all the help and encouragement they can get to stick with it . . . rewards are one important way to do this.

How to Build an Effective Reward System

When working together to build an effective reward system, here are some points to keep in mind:

- A behavioral reward system is more effective when you and your child work collaboratively to develop a list of rewards. This allows your child to identify what is motivating to them, and they will value the system since they helped develop it.
- Brainstorming a list of all possible rewards is a good first step. Parents, suspend your judgment until the list is complete! Afterwards, those ideas that are not practical, reasonable, or feasible can be removed or altered.

(page 2 of 4)

- Families are more likely to stick with a rewards program if they use charts for tracking OCD homework and associated rewards.
- Rewards must follow rather than precede behaviors.
- Rewards are most effective when they are given soon after the behavior. A reward that a child must wait all week to receive will very quickly lose its appeal.
- Rewards must be something special. They are not effective if you were going to give them to your child anyway.
- Rewards generally need to be small and relatively inexpensive. Alternatively, tokens can be earned toward a bigger reward.
- Rewards should be proportional to the level of challenge. In other words, little rewards for small ERP challenges, bigger rewards for bigger and more challenging ERPs.
- Rewards should be given for attempting or completing a task, not for a perfect performance. They are also not given for reporting decreases in anxiety, as this can lead to false reports of symptom improvement.

Reward Suggestions

Not every reward is going to be motivating for every child. What appeals to a 10-year-old will not appeal to a 16-year-old. Your child will know what rewards they would be willing to work for. Here is a list of reward suggestions that have been successfully used by other families in our program.

Age	Reward
Young children	Stickers, gum, bubbles, Hershey kisses/gummy bears/small candies, temporary tattoos, privileges, special time with parents, access to reserved toys (e.g., electronic gaming system)
Elementary school	Special activities (e.g., local pool, climbing gym), toys, screen time, time alone with parents and without siblings
Preteen	Screen time, access to desired activities, apps, gift cards, $$$, privileges
High school	Gas cards, gift cards, access to the car, apps, texting time, later curfew, $$$, privileges

In some families, children have free and complete access to computers, TV, cell phones, toys, and so forth. In other words, it can be hard for children to earn extra privileges if they already have access to everything. In those cases, it may be necessary for families to implement some limits so that children have something to work toward. Your therapist can help you problem-solve this barrier when trying to set up a reward system.

Common Questions about Reward Programs

"Isn't this bribing my child to work on their OCD?"

No, a reward system is about acknowledging the effort the child has made to address the OCD so that they will be more motivated to do the same again in the future. Remember, a reward comes after the behavior, whereas a bribe comes before.

"Shouldn't my child have enough motivation to do ERPs without rewards?"

Your child is motivated to deal with the OCD. They demonstrate that by showing up for their sessions. The treatment for OCD requires a lot of hard work that is often uncomfortable, even initially terrifying, for children. It is a lot to expect children to embrace the treatment with open arms. Sometimes a reward system can move the treatment process along, as children have some additional motivators to encourage them to do homework, practice ERPs, etc. Remember, there aren't too many adults who would show up to work if we weren't being paid . . . isn't a salary the biggest reward system of all?

"Isn't this going to be really expensive?"

Rewards do not have to be costly. Rewards may include "special time" between a parent and a child or a special privilege such as choosing what will be for dinner. You would be surprised at how easily motivated children are by small token rewards. If finances are a concern, consider placing greater emphasis on privileges rather than on material items. No matter the type of reward your child is motivated by, remember this: Any reward system is going to be cheaper than a lifetime of OCD.

"Am I going to have to reward my child forever?"

No. In fact, a good reward system also has a plan for discontinuation. Over time, as your child experiences success and is rewarded for their efforts, you will begin to scale back on the rewards such that they have to do more to get the same rewards. For example, if your child initially earned an extra 30 minutes of screen time for doing one ERP, they will soon be required to complete two ERPs in order to earn that same additional screen time. With each success, your child's internal motivation will grow, and over time, external rewards will no longer be necessary. But praise and encouragement from parents is always required!

"What if my child isn't motivated by rewards?"

It is incredibly rare for a child not to be motivated at least in some way by a behavioral reward system. If this strategy isn't working for you, it's most likely because the particular rewards being used are not motivating for your child (or are being delivered after too long a delay). Sometimes parents and children need to be creative and think outside the box to generate reward ideas. For some children with "scrupulosity" OCD symptoms (that is, marked concern with morality, fairness, and selflessness), they may initially refuse all rewards. One approach that can help in such cases is to contribute a certain amount toward a charity of their choice for attempting an ERP challenge.

(page 4 of 4)

> MODULE 2 HANDOUTS AND WORKSHEETS FOR PARENTS

Parent Homework for Module 2

For homework in this module, sit down with your child and develop a behavioral reward program using the charts provided. Also complete the Parent Monitoring worksheet and the Therapist Update.

Brainstorm a List of Rewards for Bossing Back OCD

Initially try to have some fun by brainstorming rewards with your child. At this point try to reserve judgment and indulge your child in "wishful thinking." This can be an opportunity for building your child's motivation and enthusiasm—the sky is the limit! Unrealistic rewards can be discarded later.

_____
_____
_____
_____
_____
_____
_____

Establish a Parent–Child Contract

ERP _____

_____

Reward _____

ERP _____

_____

Reward _____

ERP _____

_____

Reward _____

ERP _____

_____

Reward _____

From *OCD in Children and Adolescents: The "OCD Is Not the Boss of Me" Manual* by Katherine McKenney, Annie Simpson, and S. Evelyn Stewart. Copyright © 2020 The Guilford Press. Permission to photocopy this material is granted to purchasers of this book for personal use or use with children or youth and their parents (see copyright page for details). Purchasers can download additional copies of this material, in color (see the box at the end of the table of contents).

MODULE 2 HANDOUTS AND WORKSHEETS FOR PARENTS

Parent Monitoring for Module 2

Each week, monitor the OCD behaviors you observe. These include specific rituals (for example, handwashing, checking), things your child avoids doing, and any OCD-related accommodations that your child requires. Estimate how often these behaviours occur per day and record your response to them (that is your emotional and/or behavioral reaction). Please bring this sheet with you to the next session.

OCD behaviors (compulsions/avoidance/demands)	Estimated daily average	Parental response

---

From *OCD in Children and Adolescents: The "OCD Is Not the Boss of Me" Manual* by Katherine McKenney, Annie Simpson, and S. Evelyn Stewart. Copyright © 2020 The Guilford Press. Permission to photocopy this material is granted to purchasers of this book for personal use or use with children or youth and their parents (see copyright page for details). Purchasers can download additional copies of this material, in color (see the box at the end of the table of contents).

MODULE 2 HANDOUTS AND WORKSHEETS FOR PARENTS

Therapist Update for Module 2
(to bring to the next session)

Describe any new symptoms that you noticed over the past week:

_____
_____
_____
_____
_____

Describe any particularly challenging OCD situations that occurred over the week:

_____
_____
_____
_____
_____

Describe any successes that your child experienced over the week:

_____
_____
_____
_____
_____

Is there anything else that you think your child's therapist needs to know about the past week? If so, please describe:

_____
_____
_____
_____
_____

From *OCD in Children and Adolescents: The "OCD Is Not the Boss of Me" Manual* by Katherine McKenney, Annie Simpson, and S. Evelyn Stewart. Copyright © 2020 The Guilford Press. Permission to photocopy this material is granted to purchasers of this book for personal use or use with children or youth and their parents (see copyright page for details). Purchasers can download additional copies of this material, in color (see the box at the end of the table of contents).

MODULE 3

Foundational Treatment Tools

Breaking Free of OCD's Traps, Bossing Back OCD, and Identifying Family Accommodation

The treatment materials presented in Module 3 are designed to help children and youth shift their interpretations of their obsessions and respond differently to their intrusive thoughts. We introduce the concept of the OCD trap as something that strengthens the cycle of obsessions, uncomfortable feelings (e.g., anxiety, distress, disgust, "not right"), and compulsions. Children are also taught how to talk back to the OCD rather than perpetuate this cycle. Just as youth gain a better understanding of how this cycle is strengthened through negative reinforcement, parents also gain a better understanding of how they may be inadvertently reinforcing OCD through parental accommodations.

OCD's Trap

The concept of OCD's trap is used to help youth understand how they become stuck doing things they don't want to do, and that often don't make sense. Help your client lay out how obsessional triggers (e.g., touching a doorknob in public) result in obsessions (e.g., "It's covered in germs"; "I might throw up"), uncomfortable emotions (e.g., anxiety or distress), compulsions (e.g., using hand sanitizer), and temporary relief. While it is helpful for therapists to understand that OCD's trap is maintained through negative reinforcement, it's more important for the child or youth and their parents to realize that compulsions alleviate negative emotions temporarily, which makes it more likely that they will engage in the same behavior the next time they are bothered by an intrusive thought. Help them to understand that completing rituals never gives them a chance to realize that the feared outcome won't come true (or if it does, that they are able to cope with their distress without doing rituals). For those struggling with more feeling-based obsessions (e.g., just doesn't feel right), completing rituals also does not give them the opportunity to see that the uncomfortable feelings will pass on their own.

Once these concepts have been taught, therapists can now introduce the idea of breaking free from the OCD bully's trap by responding with more realistic and helpful cognitions. This is not the same as cognitive restructuring. In fact, we usually want to actively avoid this kind of cognitive technique, as outlining the evidence that supports or refutes the feared outcome can become a ritual itself. When escaping the OCD bully's trap, the child or youth is encouraged to develop a few brief statements or coping thoughts that challenge the intrusive obsession. We also introduce the idea that OCD is a liar and one can't trust what it says.

Bossing Back the OCD Bully

OCD can make it almost impossible for affected children and youth to act reasonably in certain situations, even if they know, for example, that they won't really turn into someone else if they walk in a "bad guy's" path or that they won't really get sick and die if they touch a specific door handle. In those situations, it can be helpful to teach kids and youth to "boss back the OCD bully." This involves teaching them how to generate some assertive and forceful statements that they can tell the OCD bully in order to show it who really is "the boss."

We will present a variety of "bossing back" statements that others have come up with. However, to be truly effective, it is important that the words be authentic to that child, using their own words and typical language. We encourage age-appropriate language, and for adolescents that may include some curse words that have more impact.

Here are some examples of bossing-back statements to present before getting the children or youth to generate their own personalized ones.

- "I don't have to listen to this bully."
- "I'm in charge, not the OCD bully."
- "If what the OCD bully told me was true, then everyone would believe it."
- "The OCD bully is a liar."
- "It's just a thought, it will pass in time."
- "Get a life, bully, this one's mine!"
- "You can keep going, OCD bully, but I'm getting off this ride!"

It is often helpful to have kids brainstorm and write out ideas on a big piece of paper and then choose the three that they feel are the most impactful for them. Once they have selected the best "boss-back" statements, they can write them on a cue card or put them into their phone to remind them of what they can say to boss back the OCD when it is bugging them.

Identifying Family Accommodations and OCD-Related Reassurance Seeking

Accommodation in the context of OCD refers to any change a family makes to their daily life in an effort to reduce the frequency, duration, or impact of their child's rituals, to relieve the anxiety and discomfort their child is experiencing in an OCD-triggered moment, or to support OCD-related avoidance.

Accommodating OCD almost always stems from a desire to reduce the affected individual's distress. Sometimes families accommodate when a child's OCD is very persuasive (or even coercive). Other times, families may not even be aware of their accommodations. It is critical that the extent of accommodation be assessed and directly addressed in therapy. If not, the hard work conducted in sessions may be undone in the home environment.

Family accommodation often emerges as a slow but insidious process that expands in tandem with OCD severity and complexity. As a child or youth's symptoms worsen, the degree of accommodation tends to increase. It is not unusual for parents to observe themselves giving in to OCD by doing things that they realize are dysfunctional. However, these acts of accommodation are often perceived as necessary to enable the family's day-to-day survival and to maintain a degree of peace in the household. The problem, of course, is that parent concession to OCD demands tends to worsen rather than improve the long-term situation. This notably contrasts with many pre-OCD parental experiences, such as providing attention and a bandage to a child's skinned knee, which would bring about resolution of the "crisis," rather than reinforcing it.

Types of Family Accommodation

Family accommodation is extremely common in OCD. Research suggests that at least 90% of families report some degree of accommodation. The types of accommodation vary, but here is a list of some illustrative examples:

1. *Facilitating rituals*
   - Buying lots of soap/hand sanitizer for washing rituals
   - Driving the car back to the house to check that the doors are locked
2. *Facilitating avoidance*
   - Taking an alternative driving route to avoid a "contaminated" area
   - Turning the taps off for the child after washing
3. *Providing reassurance*
   - Telling the child that they are not going to get sick
   - Telling the child that they are not going to act on their feared impulse
4. *Giving in to ritual-related demands*
   - Whispering so that the child's prayers aren't interrupted
   - Wearing socks in the house so that the floor doesn't get "contaminated"
5. *Decreasing the child's day-to-day responsibilities*
   - The child no longer has to do laundry because of contamination fears
   - The child no longer has to clean the bathroom because of fears of cleansers
6. *Participating in rituals*
   - Parents washing hands more than necessary
   - Checking stove burners even though they are known to be turned off
7. *Refraining from saying/doing things*
   - Not entering certain areas of the house
   - Avoiding talk about topics related to child's obsessions

8. *Waiting for the child*
   - Waiting for the child to finish a ritual before leaving the house
9. *Modifying the family routine*
   - Changing how often the garbage is taken out
   - Doing excessive loads of laundry
   - Modifying sleeping arrangements

CASE EXAMPLE

At their first appointment, Hailey and her parents describe quite different stories related to the impacts and severity of her OCD. All three agree that she does indeed have OCD, related to her fear of being responsible for "something disastrous" happening to their family. Hailey reports that she does not want to engage in ERP or other treatment for OCD because "It's just not that bad—we are doing okay." Her parents look desperate, exasperated, and stressed, stating that they "can't take it anymore." On further questioning, it emerges that Hailey has been sending texts to her parents approximately 10 times per hour when away from home, insisting that they check to make sure she hasn't left an iron plugged in, the stove or dishwasher turned on, a door unlocked, etc. If they do not reply, she continues to text and call incessantly, and subsequently returns home to check herself. Due to Hailey's distress when having these thoughts away from home, her parents agreed last year that she could quit soccer and installed online cameras in the kitchen and her bedroom to check for dangers via iPhone. She has been sleeping on her parents' bedroom floor, as she's worried that she could not rescue them quickly enough from her bedroom in case of a fire in the middle of the night. Her parents have learned that the evening news should not be watched, in case there is a story about house fires. In fact, the word *fire* is now forbidden in Hailey's presence. She has been relieved from dishwasher duties. Her routines of checking all appliances, etc., before leaving home have become more complex and now last up to 2 hours, meaning that she (and the parent driving her) were late for school or work over many months. Most recently, Hailey switched to an at-home schooling program, and her mother has taken a leave of absence from work to support this.

The above example is a composite of commonly reported histories in OCD-affected families. This includes parent facilitation and participation in rituals (checking stove, etc.) and avoidance (Hailey quitting soccer, then school), provision of reassurance (in texts, calls, and in person) and other OCD-related demands (buying in-home cameras), decreasing child responsibilities (dishwasher duties), refraining from saying things (e.g., the word *fire*), waiting (to bring Hailey to school), and modifying the family routine (Hailey sleeping on her parents' bedroom floor).

Parents often find themselves struggling to balance the perceived need to protect their child from OCD-related anxiety against the need to push the child to face their fears and refrain from performing compulsive rituals. The best course of action is to address this with a message that incorporates both ideas into a single message of support for the child. In other words, it is best for parents to acknowledge their child's distress while simultaneously directing them toward appropriate (non-OCD) strategies to cope with that distress.

Teach the parents to use statements such as the following:

- "This is tough, but I know you can get through it."
- "I know this is a hard situation, but you can learn to manage it."
- "OCD is being bossy, but I know you can do this."
- "It's my job to help you cope with the OCD, and that's not by giving into it."

Although much of the focus on accommodations tends to be on actions of the parents, they are rarely the only family members involved. Siblings are often asked to modify daily routines or behaviors to reduce the chances of triggering OCD-related distress or rituals. Friends and teachers are also asked to help with rituals at school or to facilitate avoidance of obsessional triggers. As the therapist, it is essential to look out for and address any accommodations. The next module will focus on helping parents pull back on the accommodations.

Homework Assignments

For Module 3, therapists can assign the following for youth and parents to complete at home before the next session:

For Youth

- Complete the OCD Bully's Trap Home Practice worksheet.
- Practice at least two ERPs daily between sessions. These ERPs are developed in session and recorded on the ERP Home Practice for Module 3 worksheet.

For Parents

- Complete the Parent Monitoring worksheet (parent observations of various compulsions, avoidance behaviors, and accommodations that the child requires, as well as estimated per-day average of each, and how parents responded).
- Complete the OCD Accommodation Tracking form.
- Complete the Therapist Update worksheet. This worksheet allows parents to share with the child's therapist any new OCD symptoms that were observed over the week, any particularly challenging OCD situations the family encountered, any successes the child experienced, and any other information parents feel would be helpful for the therapist to know. Therapists should ask parents to provide them with this completed worksheet at the start of the next session so they can address specific issues as needed with the child or with the whole family together.

MODULE 3 HANDOUTS AND WORKSHEETS FOR CHILDREN OR YOUTH

Breaking Free from the OCD Bully's Trap

So far we've been learning about the behaviors and feelings associated with OCD. Now it's time to focus more on the thoughts.

Cognitive-behavioral therapy (CBT), which is what you're doing in this program, is based on the idea that, in any situation, your thoughts, feelings, and behaviors are all connected. How you *think* about a situation affects how you *feel* and how you *act*. In terms of OCD, your obsessions (thoughts) affect how you feel, which causes you to do compulsions or rituals (behaviors).

So how does OCD convince you to spend so much time doing strange and silly things that you know don't make sense? It's because you've been lured into the OCD bully's trap!

When an obsession pops into your head, you start to worry. This worry thought is unpleasant, and it makes you feel stressed, anxious, or just plain yucky. You want to make the feelings stop so you do a compulsion or ritual, which makes you feel better for a little while. The problem is that the next time an obsession pops up, you'll need to do more compulsions in order to feel better . . . before you know it, you're stuck in the OCD bully's trap!

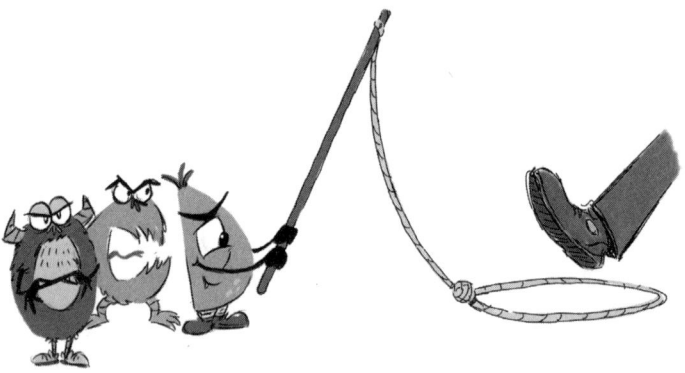

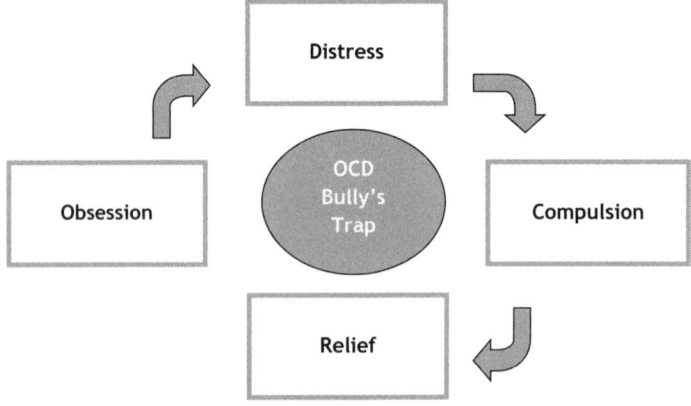

(page 1 of 5)

From *OCD in Children and Adolescents: The "OCD Is Not the Boss of Me" Manual* by Katherine McKenney, Annie Simpson, and S. Evelyn Stewart. Copyright © 2020 The Guilford Press. Permission to photocopy this material is granted to purchasers of this book for personal use or use with children or youth and their parents (see copyright page for details). Purchasers can download additional copies of this material, in color (see the box at the end of the table of contents).

Once you're in the OCD bully's trap, it can be really hard to stop doing your compulsions. That's because the compulsions do make you feel better. The OCD bully tricks you into thinking that doing compulsions is the only way to make the obsessions and bad feelings go away. He's lying! He doesn't tell you that this relief is only temporary and that over time, you'll need to do more and more compulsions to get the same temporary relief.

It's also hard to stop compulsions because the idea of not doing them feels really bad. Kids worry that the bad thing they fear will come true if they don't do the ritual. Often they fear that they won't be able to cope with their worry, or that the worry will never go away. The OCD bully doesn't give you the opportunity to discover that your fears won't come true or learn that the bad feelings and worries will fade in time.

How are *you* getting stuck in the OCD bully's trap? Pick an obsession and describe how it makes you feel, what you do to make the thought go away (compulsion), and how you feel after the compulsion.

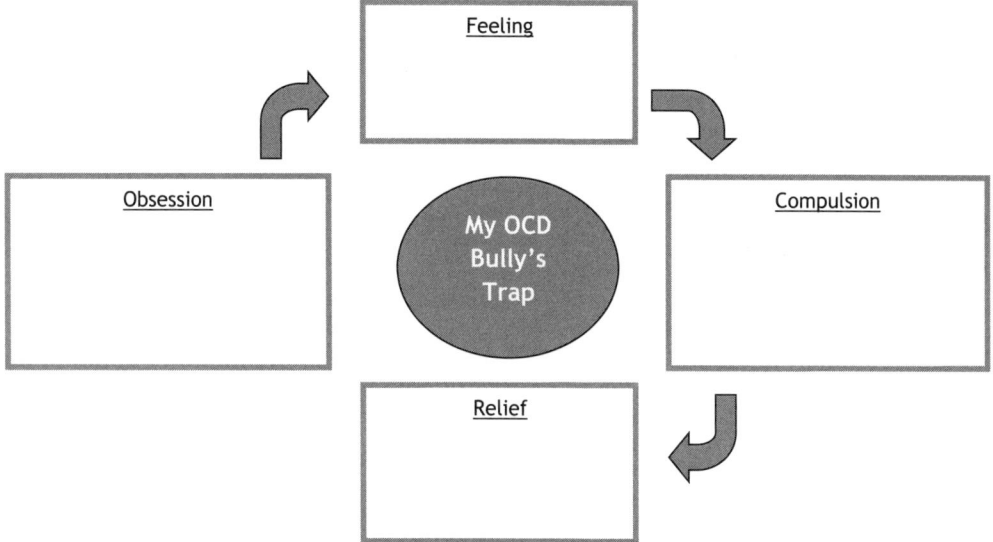

So how do we break free from this OCD bully's trap? If you are able to change just one part of this trap, you will start to break free from the Bully's grasp. We've already started to work on changing your compulsions through ERP, so we're going to spend today learning about how we can challenge the lies that the OCD bully tells you. When we're able to start thinking differently, we'll start feeling differently and acting differently too. In the case of OCD, that means feeling less anxious, or stressed, or grossed out, and doing fewer compulsions.

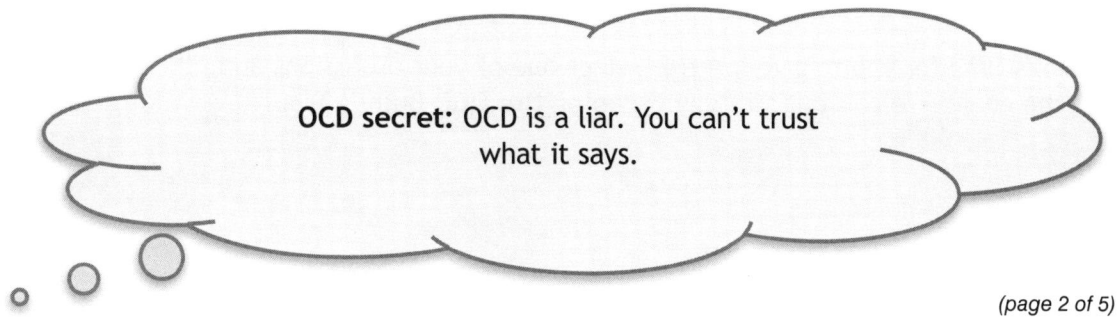

OCD secret: OCD is a liar. You can't trust what it says.

(page 2 of 5)

Let's look at an example of an OCD bully's trap and how you can challenge the Bully's lies. Imagine you're doing your homework and you wrote down the number 3, which is a problem for you:

Situation: Sitting at my desk in my room, working on my math homework

Feelings:
Stressed, Anxious, Scared

Obsession

I just wrote the number 3, which is an unlucky number. Now something bad might happen to my mom. I better fix this before she gets hurt.

OCD Bully's Trap

Compulsion/Avoidance

Tap the wall five times to prevent something bad from happening to my mother.

To change how we feel and act in a situation, we need to start thinking differently about what the OCD bully is telling us and develop our own, more realistic thoughts. Let's see what this looks like when we escape from the OCD bully's trap:

Feelings:
Calmer, less anxious

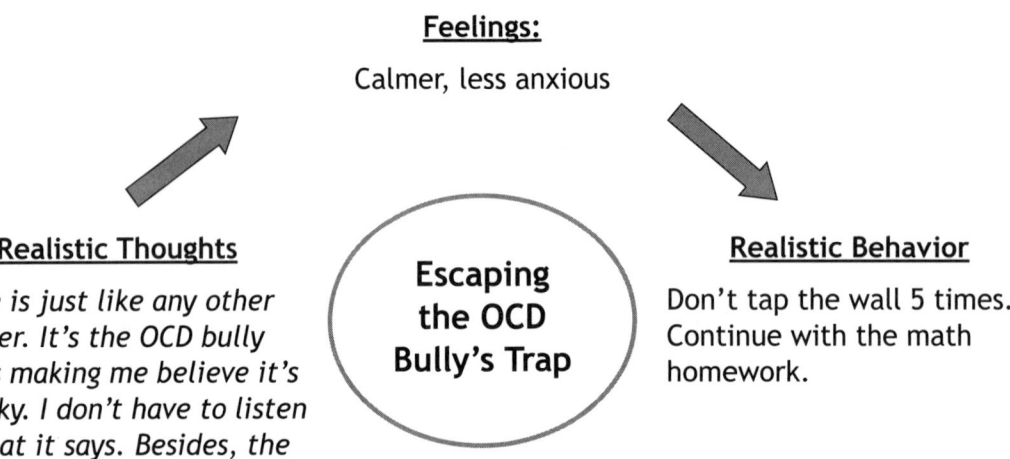

Realistic Thoughts

Three is just like any other number. It's the OCD bully that's making me believe it's unlucky. I don't have to listen to what it says. Besides, the number 3 and my mom's safety aren't related.

Escaping the OCD Bully's Trap

Realistic Behavior

Don't tap the wall 5 times. Continue with the math homework.

Now it's time for you to give it a try. Select one of your obsessions and fill out the chart. We call this strategy **Escaping the OCD Bully's Trap**.

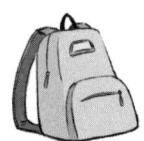

(page 3 of 5)

Situation: _____

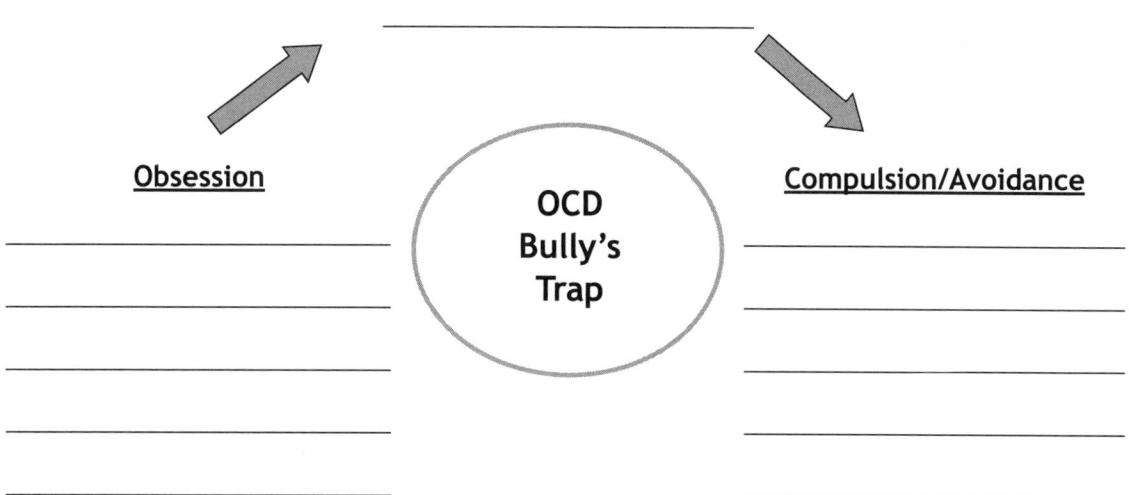

Now try breaking free from the OCD bully's trap!

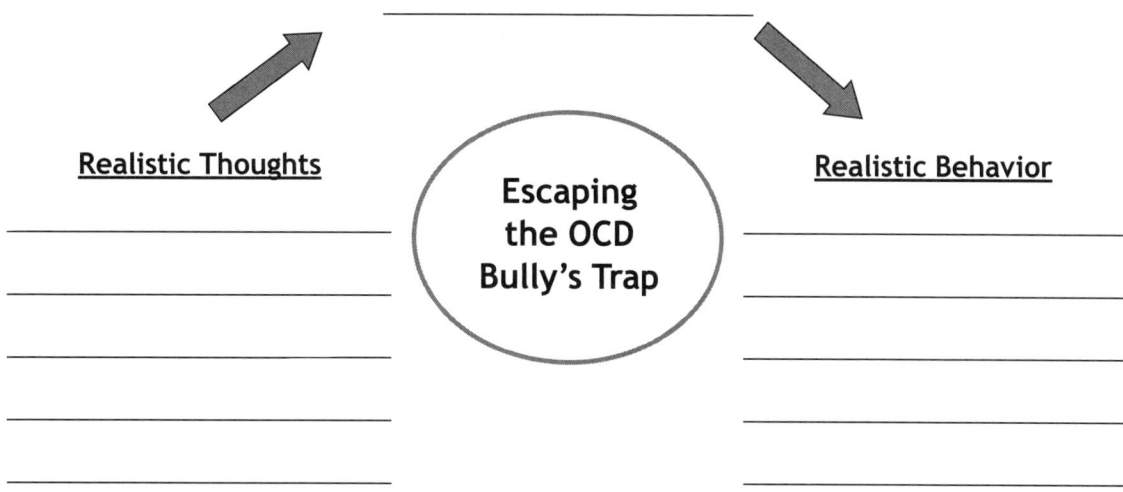

(page 4 of 5)

What if I can't think realistically about what the OCD bully is telling me?

If you're feeling really upset in an OCD moment it can be hard to think realistically about what your OCD bully is telling you. In those situations, it can be helpful to boss back the OCD bully. Each week, you and your therapist have been thinking about some things you can tell your OCD bully as part of your homework. You didn't realize it, but you were already using a strategy: **Boss Back the OCD Bully.** Here are some other things you can say to boss back your OCD:

- I don't have to listen to this bully.
- I'm in charge, not the OCD bully.
- If what the OCD bully told me was true, then everyone would believe it.
- The OCD bully is a liar.
- It's just a thought, it will pass in time.
- Get a life, bully, this one's mine!
- You can keep going, OCD bully, but I'm getting off this ride!
- If my friend wouldn't believe this, then I don't need to believe it either.

What else can you say to boss back the OCD bully?

_____
_____
_____
_____

Great work today! Keep it up. Next time we're going to focus on how to break OCD's rules!

MODULE 3 HANDOUTS AND WORKSHEETS FOR CHILDREN OR YOUTH

The OCD Bully's Trap Home Practice

Situation: _____

Feelings: _____

Obsession

_____
_____
_____
_____
_____

OCD Bully's Trap

Compulsion/Avoidance

_____
_____
_____
_____
_____

Now try breaking free from the OCD bully's trap!

Feelings: _____

Realistic Thoughts

_____
_____
_____
_____
_____

Escaping the OCD Bully's Trap

Realistic Behavior

_____
_____
_____
_____
_____

From *OCD in Children and Adolescents: The "OCD Is Not the Boss of Me" Manual* by Katherine McKenney, Annie Simpson, and S. Evelyn Stewart. Copyright © 2020 The Guilford Press. Permission to photocopy this material is granted to purchasers of this book for personal use or use with children or youth and their parents (see copyright page for details). Purchasers can download additional copies of this material, in color (see the box at the end of the table of contents).

MODULE 3 HANDOUTS AND WORKSHEETS FOR CHILDREN OR YOUTH

ERP Home Practice for Module 3

ERP task	Goal for the week	Daily homework results
		Day 1:
		Day 2:
		Day 3:
		Day 4:
		Day 5:
		Day 6:
	Reward:	Day 7:
		Day 1:
		Day 2:
		Day 3:
		Day 4:
		Day 5:
		Day 6:
	Reward:	Day 7:

From *OCD in Children and Adolescents: The "OCD Is Not the Boss of Me" Manual* by Katherine McKenney, Annie Simpson, and S. Evelyn Stewart. Copyright © 2020 The Guilford Press. Permission to photocopy this material is granted to purchasers of this book for personal use or use with children or youth and their parents (see copyright page for details). Purchasers can download additional copies of this material, in color (see the box at the end of the table of contents).

MODULE 3 HANDOUTS AND WORKSHEETS FOR PARENTS

Identifying Family Accommodation

As your child begins to make progress with ERPs, it is important that parents have a better understanding of family accommodation and are able to identify ways in which your family may be inadvertently reinforcing your child's OCD.

The focus of your child's treatment session is on cognitive strategies. In other words, we focus on identifying the faulty assumptions that underlie obsessions and learn to challenge these ideas by developing more realistic and evidence-based thoughts. In order to first identify these faulty assumptions (which often have to do with overestimations of danger and responsibility), it helps to better understand the role of obsessions in OCD

Review of Material Covered in the Module 3 Handouts and Worksheets for Children or Youth

The following concepts are presented:

OCD trap: The OCD trap is used to explain the cycle of obsessions, distress, and compulsions.
OCD Trap

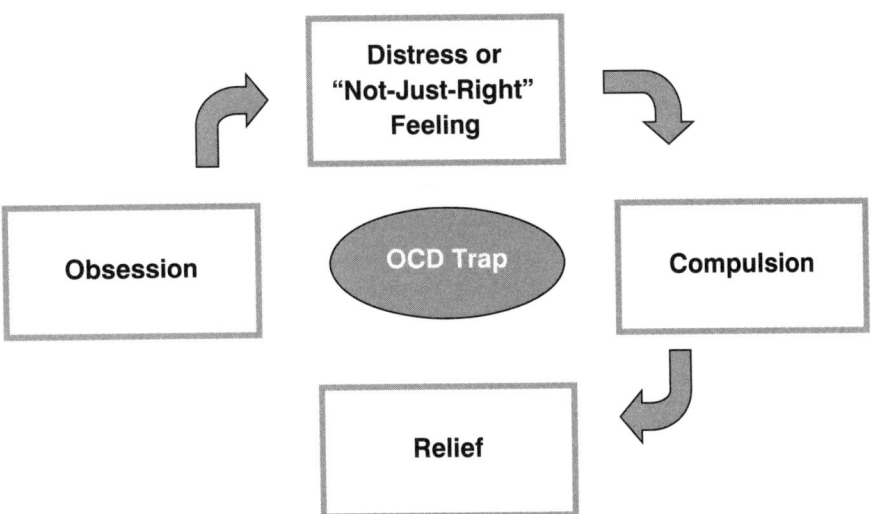

When your child encounters an obsessional trigger (for example, touching a doorknob in public), they are plagued by intrusive obsessions (for example, "It's covered in germs. I'm going to get sick). The thoughts make your child feel anxious, uncomfortable, or even disgusted. To alleviate these feelings, your child engages in a compulsion (for example, handwashing). Doing so temporarily alleviates the anxiety, which helps the intrusive thought fade. This trap is maintained through the process of negative reinforcement. That is, the compulsion removes an uncomfortable feeling so your child is reinforced to continue engaging in this behavior. It is very difficult to interrupt this process of negative reinforcement. Many children believe that

(page 1 of 4)

From *OCD in Children and Adolescents: The "OCD Is Not the Boss of Me" Manual* by Katherine McKenney, Annie Simpson, and S. Evelyn Stewart. Copyright © 2020 The Guilford Press. Permission to photocopy this material is granted to purchasers of this book for personal use or use with children or youth and their parents (see copyright page for details). Purchasers can download additional copies of this material, in color (see the box at the end of the table of contents).

their feared outcome will come true or that the uncomfortable feelings they experience will never fade. This process also does not give your child the opportunity to discover that these are mistaken beliefs.

In order for your child to free themselves from the OCD Trap, they need to start changing one of the components. The process of ERPs helps to target the compulsions/avoidance. The focus of today's session is to develop more realistic and helpful thoughts to counter the obsessional fears. This strategy is referred to as "escaping the OCD bully's trap."

Boss back the OCD bully: Another way to address obsessions is to use a strategy called "boss back the OCD." This is a form of self-talk in which the child refuses to give in to OCD and talks back to it in a forceful manner. These types of statements help children to externalize the OCD (that is, see it as something outside of themselves) and build their confidence and motivation to tackle it. Rather than challenging specific obsessions (for example, "My house won't burn down if I don't check the stove"), bossing back the OCD involves more general statements, such as these:

- "I don't have to listen to OCD."
- "I'm in charge, not OCD."
- "If what OCD told me was true, then everyone would believe it."
- "OCD is a liar."
- "I'm not falling for this, OCD. Better luck next time!"

Exposure and Response Prevention (ERP) for Parents

Before we talk about family accommodation, try this experiential exercise in order to better understand the challenges your child faces when doing an ERP, while remembering that ERPs are the treatment of choice for OCD. As contamination fears in OCD are very common, our first ERP involves picking out a jellybean (or unwrapped candy) from an open jar and then following these directions:

- First make mental notes of the level of your anxiety, or disgust, or discomfort (0–10) throughout the exercise.
- Lick the candy and then rub it under the table where you are sitting, perhaps thinking about how rarely the underside of this table is cleaned.
- Lick it again and rub it on the floor. Note the level of your anxiety, or disgust, or discomfort.
- Lick it again and then rub it on top of your shoe or foot.
- Lick it one last time and rub it on the sole of your shoe.
- Eat the contaminated jellybean and note your level of anxiety, or disgust, or discomfort.

Think about your feelings doing this exercise. It may be helpful to keep in mind that whatever the potential risks of eating contaminated candy are, the risk of not treating OCD is likely to have a higher impact on your child being able to live a normal life.

Family Accommodation

Family accommodation refers to behaviors or changes that families make to their daily lives in an effort to:

- reduce the frequency/duration of the rituals their child is engaging in
- relieve the anxiety their child is experiencing
- reduce the impact the OCD is having on their child's ability to function normally

Accommodating OCD usually stems from a good place, such as a desire to reduce a child's distress. Sometimes families accommodate because a child's OCD is very persuasive (or even coercive). Other times, families may not even be aware of the impact of accommodations on a child's OCD.

Family accommodation is generally a slow but insidious process that develops in tandem with the OCD . . . as your child's symptoms worsen, the degree of accommodation increases. It is not unusual for parents to find themselves giving in to OCD by doing things that they realize are dysfunctional; however, these acts of accommodation enable the family to manage day-to-day tasks and maintain a degree of peace in the household. The problem, of course, is that the more a parent gives in to OCD's demands, the more demanding it tends to get.

Family accommodation is extremely common in OCD. Research suggests that at least 90% of families report at least some degree of accommodation. And this accommodation can occur in both subtle and not-so-subtle ways. Here are a few examples of the many forms of accommodation that can occur in families:

1. **Facilitate rituals**

    For example, buying lots of soap/hand sanitizer for washing rituals

    For example, driving the car back to the house to check that the doors are locked.

2. **Facilitate avoidance**

    For example, taking an alternate driving route to avoid "contaminated" area

    For example, parents turning the taps off for their child after washing

3. **Provide reassurance**

    For example, telling your child they are not going to get sick

    For example, telling your child they are not going to act on their feared impulse

4. **Give in to your child's ritual-related demands**

    For example, whispering so that the child's prayers aren't interrupted

    For example, always wearing socks in the house so that the floor doesn't get contaminated by bare feet

5. **Decrease your child's day-to-day responsibilities**

    For example, the child no longer having to do laundry because of contamination fears

    For example, the child no longer having to clean the bathroom because of fears of cleansers

6. **Participate in rituals**

    For example, washing your hands more than necessary

    For example, checking stove burners even though you know they are off

(page 3 of 4)

7. **Refrain from saying/doing things**

    For example, not entering certain areas of the house

    For example, avoidance of topics related to child's obsessions

8. **Wait for your child**

    For example, waiting for your child to finish a ritual before you can leave the house for work or school

9. **Modify the family routine**

    For example, changing how often the garbage is taken out

Parents often find themselves struggling to balance the need to protect their child from anxiety with pushing them to face their fears and not give in to rituals. The best course of action is one that incorporates both ideas into a single message of support. In other worse, it's best when parents can acknowledge their child's distress while simultaneously directing them toward increased coping with that distress. The following statements incorporate these combined ideas:

- "This is tough but I know you can get through this."
- "I know this is a hard situation, but you can learn to manage it."
- "OCD is being bossy, but I'm sure you'll be okay."
- "It's my job to help you cope with the OCD."

Although we tend to focus on accommodations made by parents, they often aren't the only family members who give in to OCD. Siblings are often asked to modify daily routines or behaviors to reduce the chances of triggering the OCD. Sometimes friends are asked to help with rituals at school or to facilitate avoidance of obsessional triggers (for example, complete tasks for your child). Eventually, all forms of accommodation will need to be tackled, but for now, let's start with accommodations at home.

Next time, we will focus on how to start setting limits on these behaviors. Just as your child is using a gradual approach to face their fears, parents must use a similar approach when pulling back on accommodations. Before you start withdrawing accommodation, however, you first need to develop a greater awareness of how and when it occurs. Once that is complete, the next step is to acknowledge it. For example, if your child repeatedly asks you for reassurance, try acknowledging it in the following way:

"That is the OCD bully speaking. For now, I will go along with your request, but as you get better at taking charge of OCD, I will be on your side fighting the OCD bully's demands and refusing to go along with it."

Over time you will be talking to your child about when and how you will be refusing to go along with OCD. This is often best done with your child and therapist in the meetings where specific ERPs are discussed. It is a process of collaborative negotiation. Next time, we will spend more time discussing how to do this.

For homework, use the OCD Accommodation Tracking form to monitor the different types of accommodations as they occur throughout the day. This form will help you figure out what accommodations to tackle first.

MODULE 3 HANDOUTS AND WORKSHEETS FOR PARENTS

Parent Monitoring for Module 3

Each week, monitor the OCD behaviors you observe. These include specific rituals (for example, handwashing, checking), things your child avoids doing, and any OCD-related accommodations your child requires. Estimate how often these occur per day and record your response to them (that is, your emotional and/or behavioral reaction). Please bring this sheet with you to the next session.

OCD behaviors (compulsions/avoidance/demands)	Estimated daily average	Parental response

From *OCD in Children and Adolescents: The "OCD Is Not the Boss of Me" Manual* by Katherine McKenney, Annie Simpson, and S. Evelyn Stewart. Copyright © 2020 The Guilford Press. Permission to photocopy this material is granted to purchasers of this book for personal use or use with children or youth and their parents (see copyright page for details). Purchasers can download additional copies of this material, in color (see the box at the end of the table of contents).

MODULE 3 HANDOUTS AND WORKSHEETS FOR PARENTS

Parent Homework for Module 3: OCD Accommodation Tracking

Family activity impacted by OCD	**Frequency** (for example, daily, weekly)	**Accommodation** (for example, checking for child, waiting, reassuring)	**Person accommodating** (for example, mother, father, sibling, friend)
Morning routine (for example, getting dressed)			
Arrival at school/work (for example, getting in car)			
Mealtimes (for example, specific foods, individuals permitted)			
Bedtime routines (for example, saying good night)			
Social/family functions (for example, playdates, dinner with grandparents)			
Going to restaurants			
Shopping			
Keeping appointments			
Trips/vacations			
Planning/scheduling			
Religious/spiritual worship			
Others (for example, soccer practice)			

Adapted from the OCD Family Functioning Scale, Part 1 (Stewart et al., 2011).

From *OCD in Children and Adolescents: The "OCD Is Not the Boss of Me" Manual* by Katherine McKenney, Annie Simpson, and S. Evelyn Stewart. Copyright © 2020 The Guilford Press. Permission to photocopy this material is granted to purchasers of this book for personal use or use with children or youth and their parents (see copyright page for details). Purchasers can download additional copies of this material, in color (see the box at the end of the table of contents).

MODULE 3 HANDOUTS AND WORKSHEETS FOR PARENTS

Therapist Update for Module 3
(to bring to the next session)

Describe any new symptoms that you noticed over the past week:

_____
_____
_____
_____
_____

Describe any particularly challenging OCD situations that occurred over the week:

_____
_____
_____
_____
_____

Describe any successes that your child experienced over the week:

_____
_____
_____
_____
_____

Is there anything else that you think your child's therapist needs to know about the past week? If so, please describe:

_____
_____
_____
_____
_____

From *OCD in Children and Adolescents: The "OCD Is Not the Boss of Me" Manual* by Katherine McKenney, Annie Simpson, and S. Evelyn Stewart. Copyright © 2020 The Guilford Press. Permission to photocopy this material is granted to purchasers of this book for personal use or use with children or youth and their parents (see copyright page for details). Purchasers can download additional copies of this material, in color (see the box at the end of the table of contents).

MODULE 4

Breaking OCD's Rules

The Four *S*'s, Exposure Games, and Limiting Family Accommodation and Reassurance Seeking

The Four *S*'s

As discussed in past modules, ERPs require children and youth to expose themselves to scary or distressing situations and then resist performing compulsions. Clearly, the goal of not doing the compulsion at all on day 1 may be unrealistic. It is important for them to understand that what is important is that they attempt to boss back the OCD and that they not do what the OCD is telling them to do. So, if they are able to resist compulsions—that is fantastic! But more realistically, this may initially involve limiting or changing the compulsions in such a way that they begin to lessen their hold on the child or youth. This can be done both with planned ERPs or when the child unexpectedly encounters an obsessional trigger. The "OCD Is Not the Boss of Me" program provides the "Four *S*'s" as concrete tools for the children to use if they are not initially able to entirely resist performing rituals, as follows:

1. Shift it.
2. Shrink it.
3. Switch it.
4. Silly it.

Shift It

Implement a delay before engaging in compulsions. For example, wait increasingly longer periods of time before checking locks, rereading material, or rearranging/adjusting something that feels "not right."

Shrink It

Gradually decrease the frequency or total time of engagement in a ritual. For example, a child who regularly washes his hands 10 times or for 5 minutes, can aim to decrease it to eight times or to 3 minutes. For compulsions that occur repeatedly throughout the day that involve another person (e.g., asking reassurance of a parent, excessive apologizing), a child could be provided with a certain daily number of question cards or apology cards that can be traded in for answers or acknowledgment of an apology. The number of cards allotted daily can be decreased over time as the need to seek reassurance decreases.

Switch It

Switching up a compulsion, or doing it differently, is another effective way to boss back the OCD. For example, a multistep nighttime ritual could be performed backwards or in a mixed-up order. This may make the ritual less rigid and easier to resist as treatment progresses.

Silly It

Adding humor to compulsions is another way to fight back. OCD tends to send the child a message that everything is very serious and has a way of driving conflict. Finding ways to make things funny can help diminish some of OCD's perceived power. For example, a child who is fearful of stepping on cracks can do the chicken dance while purposely stepping on lines on the sidewalk. Other ideas include singing about feared outcomes in an opera voice.

CASE EXAMPLE

Matthew and his therapist had been working together to create exposures to address his perceived need to check all elements of his house before leaving to ensure the safety of his home and family. Prior to coming to therapy, Matthew would check 15 times whether the doors were locked, nine times that the stove was off, and three times that the windows were closed. If anyone talked or interrupted his ritual, he felt he had to start again from the beginning. It was often taking the family over an hour each morning to leave the house. On almost a daily basis, both Matthew and his sister were late for school and his parents were late for work. Matthew's mother was in jeopardy of losing her job. Matthew's therapist taught him the Four S's, and together they decided to integrate these strategies into his exposures. He began to shrink the number of times he would check each of the components in his home. Similarly, he began to switch up the order in which he checked these things. Finally, as the mood in the house had become quite serious and tense while everyone waited to be able to leave, the whole family (including Matthew) began to sing "Old MacDonald" as he engaged in his rituals. Matthew was able to lessen the amount of time spent in these rituals, to decrease anxiety when changing his rituals and began to feel empowered to push back further. Within a month, he was no longer checking at all.

Making ERPs Fun: Exposure Games

The key to OCD treatment success is exposure. Exposure and response prevention is the most powerful tool in the fight against OCD. ERPs, however, don't have to be serious activities. You will be asking children and youth to expose themselves to situations that are highly distressing—it's okay for you both to have a little fun while doing it! Working with children by necessity requires a fun, playful approach. We have found that integrating exposures into fun creative games is a great way to engage children and even youth in treatment. There are no limits to the ways games and fun can be incorporated into ERPs. Be creative and connect with each child or youth to explore their interests and how they like to have fun. Then use this knowledge to create "hooks" for engagement. For example, if working with a child who loves Dora the Explorer and who has contamination obsessions and washing compulsions, create a board game where Dora has to go on missions with the map and collect various pieces of garbage and contaminants in a bag to get a prize! The trick for this approach is to make sure the games are tapping into the core OCD fear and triggers. The following examples provide different ideas for games we have used that can be adapted for various ages and developmental levels:

Two Truths and a Lie

Children write down three statements on a piece of paper. Two are true and one is a lie. This can be adapted to be an exposure for a variety of symptom presentations. This works well for children with scrupulosity who worry about lying. Depending on what is triggering for the individual child, you can choose to have them never reveal which statements are true and which are lies, or you can reveal this and then act out being angry at the child or youth for lying (to trigger fears of getting in trouble). This game also works well for individuals with perfectionism, as you can have them write the statements using messy handwriting or include spelling mistakes.

Bet You Can't Touch That

Children love a game of dare! Dare each other to touch obsessional triggers of increasing "grossness" or "dirtiness" in a friendly competition. Collect coins or stickers for each dare completed, and then trade them in at the end of the session for a reward, such as candy or something from the therapist's prize box. Having the therapist model rewarding themselves can be particularly helpful for children or youth who are reluctant to accept rewards.

Make It Grosser

Select a candy and take turns making it increasingly gross. Rub the candy on "contaminated" objects and then eat it. Each person has to touch the candy to something grosser than the last person. Examples include: under the table, on your shoe, on the ground, in the garbage can, on the door handle, on the faucet. This game can easily be modified for a group setting by taking turns in a circle, with each trying to outdo the last. Eating candy as part of exposures in general is really helpful because it can't be undone, unlike, for example, contaminating hands in session which can be washed later.

Follow the Leader

In this game, everyone (child, parents, therapist) follows a leader in a line and whatever the leader does (touches something gross, dirty etc.) everyone else in the line has repeat. Once everyone in the line has completed the exposure, it is someone else's turn to be the leader. This game can be adapted for a variety of symptom presentations.

Hot Potato

This game works well for children or youth who avoid touching certain items because they fear they have become contaminated (e.g., items from school). Sitting in a circle, have them pass "contaminated objects" quickly from person to person while music is playing. When the music stops, the person holding the item is the winner and collects a small prize. Then the next round begins with a more challenging item.

Simon Says

In a similar vein, have children play Simon Says where the focus is on touching gross or dirty things: "Simon says touch the floor"; "Simon says touch the garbage can"; "Touch your nose"; etc.

This Candy Will Make Me . . .

For children or youth who are afraid of getting sick or vomiting, a fun exposure involves having them hold a candy while describing the bad outcome that will result if they eat it—for example: "This candy will make me have a stomachache": "This candy will make me feel nauseated"; "This candy will make me vomit." Subsequently, have them eat the candy.

Maybe

Uncertainty is a core aspect of OCD. It often isn't the fear (e.g. situation, item,) itself that is the core fear, but the inability to know something with 100% certainty. For example, many teens are not afraid of being gay but are afraid of the uncertainty of their sexual orientation. "How do I know for sure?"; "Maybe I am gay but am pretending to be straight. . . ." Similarly, some may have intrusive thoughts that appear bizarre (e.g., fearing that they will take on the personal characteristics of someone they bump into). They can acknowledge the bizarreness of the thought, but the uncertainty associated with the thought ("I can never be certain that it won't happen") leads them to engage in rituals, such as checking over their shoulder. Embracing the inherent uncertainty in life can be accomplished with the Maybe Game. In this game, you and the child or youth take turns coming up with statements that start with the word *maybe*. Examples include "Maybe I'm morphing into a new horrible person"; "Maybe I already am a horrible murderer who kills small animals"; "Maybe I'll get married and still not know for sure whether I'm gay"; etc. The trick is to tap into the core of whatever the child or youth is uncertain about.

"Not-Right" Feeling Game

For children who struggle with needing to get a "just-right" feeling, doing things on purpose to simulate a wrong feeling can be a fun way of doing exposures. Examples include: walking around to music with shoes on the wrong feet, writing silly statements to each other using the nondominant hand, wearing clothes inside out and/or backwards, parting hair on the wrong side of their head, etc. The purpose is to trigger a "wrong feeling" and then habituate to that. Once children have experienced how a "strong feeling" can pass, then therapists can introduce exposures that are more specifically related to the child's "not-right" OCD symptoms.

Bingo, Memory/Concentration, and Go Fish

All three of these games can be adapted to address a multitude of fears by using triggering words. For example, a memory game can be created by writing pairs of words on cards, mixing them up, and then trying to find matches. The person with the most matches wins. To make the game more effective, therapists and children should read aloud the word on the card as they flip them over. Example of words for harm-related obsessions could include *murder, kill, rape, gun, suicide, death*, etc. Similarly, a Bingo card can be created with triggering words, and the first person who completes a line yells, "Bingo!" Go Fish can be played with a goal of getting pairs of triggering words by asking each other for them—for example, do you have *vomit*?"

Scavenger Hunts, Exposure Olympics, and Mission Possible

There are many different ways to incorporate exposures into a fun race-like activity. Examples include scavenger hunts, Olympics, or "mission possible" cards where kids or youth grab a mission from an envelope and subsequently go to complete it. These games can all can be adapted to a variety of fears. Examples of exposures could include "Go touch five door handles"; "Write *cancer* in chalk four times on the sidewalk": "Go step on seven cracks in the road"; etc. With each completed exposure, the child or youth earns a piece of a puzzle, which can be assembled at the end of the game to create a picture of a specific reward.

Dare You to Do This Exposure, Exposure Revenge

This particular game works well in a group setting, particularly after children or youth are more familiar with each other's OCD symptoms. However, you can also use this game with the therapist, parents, and child all participating. Usually this results in the child developing gross challenges for parents and the therapist to do, so be prepared! Begin by writing everyone's name on a small piece of paper. Everyone draws a name and then has to create an exposure for that particular person. Take turns daring the identified person to do the exposure. The next week, introduce "Exposure Revenge," where each person has to create an exposure for the person who created one for them the previous week.

Mistakes, Break Rules Game

These games are for children or youth with scrupulosity concerns such that they are excessively rule abiding and frequently confess to minor perceived mistakes, or seek reassurance that they are doing the "right" thing. The mistakes game will help to expose them to breaking the rules. Have them go around intentionally making mistakes such as misspelling words, getting math questions wrong, or wearing their socks inside out. Similarly, an effective exposure game can be getting children or youth to break minor rules and then resist confessing in a game-like form. For example, have them litter on purpose, put recycling in the garbage, or draw minor graffiti and then not confess.

Three Good Things, Three Bad Things

The "Three Good Things, Three Bad Things" game helps children and youth to test the power of thoughts and thought–action fusion, which is when a person believes that simply thinking about an action is just as bad as actually carrying out that action. It can also lead people to believe that just thinking about an event makes it more likely that the event will occur. Have children write three good things they wish will happen to them over the week (e.g., "I wish I will win the lottery"; "I wish I will get a dog"). Then have them write three bad things they wish will happen (e.g., "I wish I will get hit by a car"; "I wish I will get cancer"). Make sure the child is selecting wishes that are plausible and possible. Have them review their wishes at the next session to see if any of them came true. This can then be used to highlight the idea that just because you wish something (or think it), it doesn't make it come true!

Goodbye and I Hope You Die

In this game, you and the child or youth take turns hoping something horrible happens to each other. This game targets those who have trouble with harm-related obsessions. You can start small with a humorous comment, and then make subsequent comments harder to say and more serious. For example, start with "Goodbye and I hope you slip on a banana peel and get eaten by a monkey." Gradually move up to more anxiety-provoking statements until you end with something like "Goodbye and I hope you get into a horrible car crash when you leave here and die a painful death." Similar to the game above, have them review their statements at the next session to see if any of them came true. This also highlights the distinction of stating something versus making it come true!

CASE EXAMPLE

Andrew was a 10-year-old boy with fears about getting sick and vomiting from exposure to germs. He was extremely avoidant of all exposures and had very little tolerance of distress.

Andrew's therapist initially worked on promoting Andrew's habituation to various trigger words by playing "goodbye and I hope you die" where all the negative outcomes involved vomiting. Andrew was able to work up to more challenging ERPs when his therapist incorporated the thing he enjoyed the most—video games. Andrew loved video games that involved creating characters doing real-life activities. He was able to create a character who resembled himself and then had the character vomit repeatedly in the toilet. Using video games made this exposure fun; however, it was still extremely challenging as it required him to watch "himself" being sick. Prior to this he was unable to even mention out loud the thought of getting sick for fear of it making it happen.

Working with Parents to Limit Accommodation

Similar to how the children are challenged to gradually decrease their rituals, it is important to challenge and work with parents to begin to limit their OCD accommodations. We should note that some parents find this much easier than others. Some parents struggle with tolerating their child's distress when OCD is triggered. It's important to limit blame between the parents about accommodations. Peris et al. (2012) found that less blame, more cohesion, and less conflict in the family predicts better CBT outcomes. The Four S's, described above, can also be used by parents in their attempts to reduce what are sometimes longstanding accommodations. Just as it's hard for children to suddenly stop rituals, it is also challenging for parents to resist accommodating OCD when seeing their child's distress. This takes practice, so remind parents to not become too discouraged when they have inadvertently or knowingly accommodated their child's OCD. Sometimes even suggesting that parents reward themselves for the hard task of pulling back on accommodations can be additionally helpful.

To do this, we first recommend selecting one target behavior at a time. The behavior chosen should be one that occurs relatively frequently, in order to provide ample opportunities for practice. Similarly, the target behavior should be a significant problem and one that the parents are motivated to address. Setting limits on accommodations will not be an easy process, as OCD will push back, especially when specific accommodations have been longstanding. A high degree of parent motivation will help keep them from giving up prematurely, and thus inadvertently reinforcing the problem. For example, choosing a target accommodation behavior such as parents doing two or three loads of laundry a day may be a more significant and motivating behavior to address than the purchasing of great quantities of hand soap. Ideally, having some degree of child "buy-in" can make the process easier. As children do not tend to readily agree to accommodation removal, offering them a choice between two accommodation types to initially address can be a useful strategy because it provides them with a sense of some control. In this circumstance it is important that the parents do not send the message that *no* accommodations will be changed, but rather that their child has some input on *which* accommodation will be first addressed.

After a target behavior has been chosen, parents will need to inform their child of the changes that will be coming. Children and youth may display a wide variety of reactions when informed that limiting of accommodations is pending. Some may be keen to receive additional support in resisting OCD; others may demonstrate no initial reaction at all. For many, the idea of reduced accommodations may trigger feelings of anxiety, distress, or even anger, which can be difficult for parents to tolerate. Regardless of their child's reaction, it is important for parents to know that in order to win the battle against OCD, parental accommodation must be addressed with or without the child's approval.

The discussion about limiting accommodations should be planned for a time when both the parent and the child or youth are relatively calm and relaxed. The therapist can play an important role in this process, most of which can transpire in the office setting.

Here are some tips to keep in mind while facilitating these discussions:

- Have parents acknowledge their child's difficulty in an empathic manner, albeit one that conveys the parents' determination and commitment to overcoming this challenge.
- Have parents focus on their own intentions, rather than those of the child. A discussion that centers around the child (e.g., "You can no longer do this . . .") will inevitably lead to arguments and noncompliance. In other words, encourage parents to use "I" statements rather than "You" statements. (e.g., "I will no longer let myself be bullied by OCD into doing your laundry two or three times a day.").
- If the child reacts in an explosive manner or if previous attempts at talking about this subject have been met with difficulties, the reader is referred to Lebowitz and Omer's (2013) book, *Treating Childhood and Adolescent Anxiety: A Guide for Caregivers* for ideas, including a written announcement to the child of the changes that will be made.

The process of setting limits on accommodations will be most effective when parents and their child work as a team. The more a child or youth is involved in the planning process, the more invested they will be in its implementation. For example, this could include inviting the child to determine how many repetitions of a question their parents will initially reply. Despite parents' best efforts to collaboratively involve their child, many children will still resist the concept of limiting accommodations. It is important that parents remain firm and resist engaging in debates or arguments around this necessary step in treatment.

Addressing OCD-Related Reassurance Seeking

As discussed throughout this book, children and youth with OCD get "sticky" thoughts in their heads that are upsetting (obsessions), and they subsequently engage in certain behaviors to alleviate their discomfort (compulsions), albeit temporarily. One subset of these compulsions that is highly prevalent in pediatric OCD is reassurance seeking from others. These others may be significant people in the child's life, such as parents, teachers, or friends, or even contacts on the Internet (e.g., online forums, online research). It could be asked, "So what, exactly, is the problem with getting reassurance?" For those without an anxiety disorder or OCD, there is little problem—in fact, this is useful behavior. A child or youth asks a trusted adult, "Is this going to make me sick?" And the adult answers, "No, you'll be fine."

The child or youth then proceeds to eat the meal that nourishes them. For most individuals, this one-time assurance is enough to allow them to continue with the task at hand.

The problem with OCD is that it creates an ongoing perceived inability of the child to tolerate uncertainty and doubt, such that one answer is not enough. OCD does not demand assurance, but demands reassurance—again and again. It introduces the notion that there is potentially something to worry about, that there must be some validity to the obsession, and that a more recent, updated answer is required. As such, the cycle of reassurance seeking begins. Unbeknownst to the parent, providing an answer (yet again) sends the message that their child must achieve some sort of certainty to be able to carry on. Yet, in reality, people continue in their lives despite the fact that very little in this world is certain.

The problem of OCD-related reassurance seeking is described in the following quotation from OCD psychotherapist Jon Hershfield:

> If reassurance were a substance, it would be considered right up there with crack cocaine. Once is never enough, a few makes you want more, tolerance is constantly on the rise, and withdrawal hurts. In other words, people with OCD and related conditions who compulsively seek reassurance get a quick fix, but actually worsen their discomfort in the long term.

The first step in assisting parents to limit reassurance provision is to explain how reassurance empowers the OCD. The parent's goal is to create the opportunity for their child to learn to tolerate distress as opposed to providing the specific answers. Families can do this by giving the child a certain number of reassurance cards to use each day. The child will be permitted a certain number of daily questions that will be answered by parents. Once these have been used, parents will respond to any additional requests for reassurance with something like the following: "Remember, I can't answer any more questions, because I don't want to feed the OCD bully; let's go do something fun together." The parent and child gradually decrease the daily number of reassurance cards provided. A fun and motivating variation on this is to decide that unused cards can be cashed in for rewards or money.

It is common for parents to get confused about what they are "allowed" to say and which questions they are "allowed" to answer. A helpful response to this situation is as follows:

> "We know from other parents that it is often confusing to figure out whether a child's particular question is OCD-related reassurance seeking (which should not be reinforced), or whether this is a reasonable question by a child to their parent (which they should probably answer as a responsible parent for teaching purposes). This is especially the case when children adamantly insist that the question isn't an OCD question.
>
> "In fact, there is no problem with asking or replying to a question once—when the parent replies in a factual manner, this is providing 'assurance.' However, if the same question (or different versions of the same question) keeps returning, it is likely that OCD is at play. Answering a question again and again is providing 'RE-assurance.' And it is not useful to debate with the child about whether or not a question is OCD related. Consensus is not required prior to limiting reassurance. However, it can be invaluable to have a discussion during a calm moment to explain to the child why this reassurance won't be given (or why it will be delayed) the next time they ask."

Examples of Accommodation Limit Setting

There are no hard-and-fast rules about how to set limits on family accommodations. The severity and nature of the OCD and the types of accommodation in place will influence how parents set limits. What follows is a list of ways to set limits for selected accommodations that emerge in the context of OCD:

1. Washing/Cleaning Rituals
   - Parents will not answer questions about their own handwashing or whether various items are contaminated.
   - Parents will not allow their child to inspect their hands for cleanliness.
   - Parents will not wash their child's clothes more frequently than other household members.
   - Parents will not purchase extra cleaning products, soap, or hand sanitizer.
2. Checking Behaviors
   - Parents will not answer questions about whether doors or windows are locked.
   - Parents will not check on their child's behalf.
   - Parents will open or unlock doors and windows as they so desire.
3. Avoidance
   - Parents will not drive via particular routes to avoid triggering the OCD.
   - Parents will not assist with the use of barriers (e.g., providing knives and forks or gloves to eat finger foods).
   - Parents will not alter household duties to enable the child to avoid OCD-triggering tasks.

Even if the child voices agreement with the plan during discussion in a calm moment, they will likely experience an increase in distress in the moment when parents limit their usual accommodation. As the therapist, it can be helpful to prepare parents for reactions of both their child and of themselves.

Once limits on accommodations have been implemented it is not uncommon for children and youth to react in challenging ways, including tantrums, screaming, damage to physical property, threats of harm, and even physical aggression toward self and others. It is important to coach parents to expect these reactions and to plan accordingly for how they will respond. Disengaging from the interaction is often an effective approach for managing the outbursts. It also ensures that parents will not be drawn into the interaction, which may prolong the behavior, exacerbate both the parents' and their child's stress, and limit everyone's ability to respond in a helpful manner. Disengaging from arguments or provocations is tricky but important, as these function to distract from the task at hand, which is to limit accommodation. It may be helpful to role-play in your office with the parents, having them practice remaining calm in situations where their child becomes highly distraught or attempts to draw them into unproductive discussions.

In some situations, it may be too difficult for parents to disengage from negative interactions while remaining in close proximity to their child. Children or youth may cling to parents, follow them around while insisting on an accommodation, or even become physically aggressive. In those instances, parents may need to physically remove themselves from the situation, presuming that their child is safe without adult supervision. This can include moving to a different location in the house, going into the backyard, sitting in their car, or leaving the premises entirely if appropriate to do so.

As progress occurs, it is important that parents continue giving positive reinforcement as their child resists OCD behavior (e.g., not asking for reassurance, reducing handwashing), and when he or she engages with the parents' attempts to limit accommodations. This does not mean that their child must be pleased by the cessation of accommodation; rather, the reinforcement should reflect the fact that their child managed to cope with the changes.

Inform parents of the potential for an extinction burst—that is, things are often likely to get worse before they get better as OCD "ups the ante" prior to succumbing to ERP.

At first, a child or youth may become very upset and anxious when their parent refuses to participate in a ritual. But over time and with repeated and consistent limit setting, they may become gradually less distressed and recover more quickly. This change reflects the child or youth's newfound ability to cope, as well as a decrease in the intensity of OCD.

Parents often relate to the following analogy that illustrates what to expect when starting to limit accommodations that have been regularly provided over a period of time:

> "Consider the situation of waiting at a checkout line in a supermarket. When your toddler sees the chocolate bars and asks for one, you shake your head 'no,' causing her to whine loudly. Although you have never agreed to this in the past, you are having a rough day and strangers are looking over disapprovingly, so you say yes. Your child smiles up at you and all is well—for the short term.
>
> "The next time you return to the store, you decide in advance that you will say no and that the others will just have to tolerate the sound of your child whining. However, when you say no on this occasion, even after her whining, she looks at you in disbelief and begins crying, flopping to the ground and kicking her arms and legs. This same scenario plays out the next three times you return to the store. Eventually she learns that, no matter what she does, she will not be able to get the chocolate bar that she so desperately wants."

In the above scenario, things get worse before they get better. The toddler represents the OCD (not the OCD-affected child), and the chocolate bar represents the accommodation that relieves or avoids the child's OCD-related distress. It takes many occasions of the parent holding their ground before the toddler refrains from "upping the ante" in an attempt to obtain their momentary need.

Homework Assignments

For Module 4, therapists can assign the following for youth and parents to complete at home before the next session.

For Youth

- Practice at least three ERPs daily between sessions. These ERPs are developed in session and recorded on the ERP Home Practice for Module 4 worksheet.

For Parents

- Complete the limiting accommodations worksheet.
- Complete the Parent Monitoring worksheet (parent observations of various compulsions, avoidance behaviors, and accommodations that the child requires, as well as estimated per-day average of each, and how parents responded).
- Complete the Therapist Update worksheet. This worksheet allows parents to share with the child's therapist any new OCD symptoms that were observed over the week, any particularly challenging OCD situations the family encountered, any successes the child experienced, and any other information parents feel would be helpful for the therapist to know. Therapists should ask parents to provide them with this completed worksheet at the start of the next session so they can address specific issues as needed with the child or with the whole family together.

MODULE 4 HANDOUTS AND WORKSHEETS FOR CHILDREN OR YOUTH

Breaking the Rules

For the past few sessions, you've been working on your ERPs for homework and with your therapist in session. You've probably been working really hard on resisting the urge to do the compulsions the OCD bully wants you to do. If you're like most kids with OCD, you have probably experienced some success, but you have also probably had some difficulties. When the OCD bully gets really bossy, it can seem impossible to ignore it or boss it back. Today we're going to learn some strategies that will help you to show the bully who is the real boss.

The OCD bully has given you lots of specific rules that it wants you to follow . . . rules like *how* you're supposed to do your rituals, *when* you need to do your rituals, *who* can be around, and so on. We're going to start breaking these rules. You have probably already started to use some of these ideas in your ERPs, so some may seem familiar, but other ideas for breaking OCD's rules may be new.

To be an OCD rule breaker, the only thing you need to remember is the letter *S* . . .

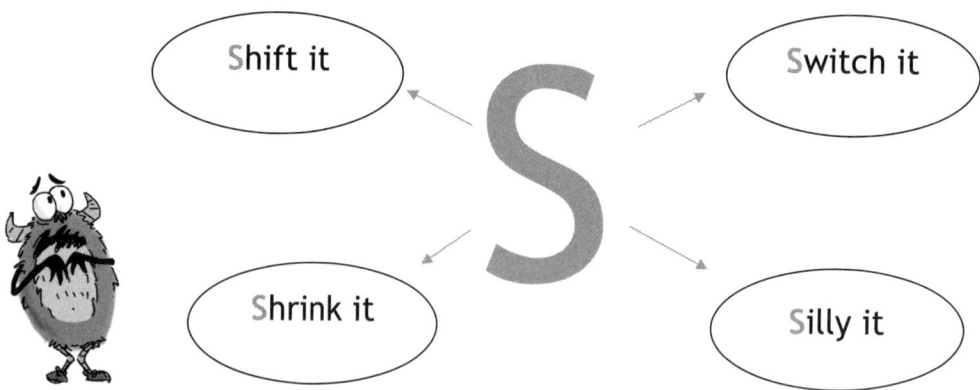

The first thing to try is to **shift it** . . . this means to shift or delay the ritual or compulsion until later. If the OCD bully is telling you to change your clothes as soon as you get home from school, try to break this rule by waiting a certain amount of time before getting changed. Start by waiting 10 or 20 minutes (or whatever you think you can handle). Each time you delay the ritual, try to go a few minutes longer. Pretty soon, you won't feel like you need to change your clothes at all because delaying the ritual allows your distress level to go down and you won't feel the pressure to do the ritual.

(page 1 of 4)

From *OCD in Children and Adolescents: The "OCD Is Not the Boss of Me" Manual* by Katherine McKenney, Annie Simpson, and S. Evelyn Stewart. Copyright © 2020 The Guilford Press. Permission to photocopy this material is granted to purchasers of this book for personal use or use with children or youth and their parents (see copyright page for details). Purchasers can download additional copies of this material, in color (see the box at the end of the table of contents).

How could you shift one of your OCD rituals until later?

_____

_____

_____

You can also try to **shrink it** . . . in other words, try to reduce the ritual in some way. If the OCD bully is telling you that you need to turn the light switch on and off 14 times, then try doing it only 10 times. Once you can manage that, try shrinking the ritual even more to 7, then 5 times. Keep reducing the number of times you need to do the ritual until you hit 0. For rituals that involve a specific amount of time (like washing your hands for 3 minutes), try shrinking the amount of time. Set the goal each day so you know what you're trying to work on.

_____

_____

_____

If the OCD bully is trying to get you to follow its rules, you can always **switch it** . . . in other words, do the ritual differently. If the OCD bully tells you to check that all the appliances are turned off in a specific order, then switch up the order. If the OCD bully tells you to reread a page, then do something else first, like watch a short YouTube video or text a friend. Do the ritual out of order, interrupt the ritual with another task, do the ritual in a different location, or only do part of the ritual . . . any of these things will show the OCD bully who is *really* in control.

How could you switch up one of your OCD rituals?

_____

_____

_____

Another way to frustrate the OCD bully is to turn the ritual into something funny. In other words, **silly it** or make it ridiculous. It's hard to be scared or anxious if you're doing something silly. So if the OCD bully is making you worry about hurting someone else, then draw a picture of yourself tickling the person with a giant feather. If the OCD bully is making you worry about stepping on cracks, then do the chicken dance while purposely walking on lines on the sidewalk. Turning your thoughts and rituals into something ridiculous will help you to annoy the OCD bully so much that he'll start to leave you alone.

(page 2 of 4)

How could you make one of your OCD rituals silly?

_____

_____

_____

Breaking the rules gives you a chance to get creative. The OCD bully has told you to do some pretty unusual and strange things, so now it's **your** turn. Think about all the ways that you can show the OCD bully who's boss. It would be great if you were able to just quit doing a ritual altogether, but for most people pushing yourself to stop something you've been doing for a long time is just too hard at first. Breaking the rules is a gradual way of resisting a compulsion.

Now it's time to break the rules! Fill out the following ERP sheet to complete in session with your therapist.

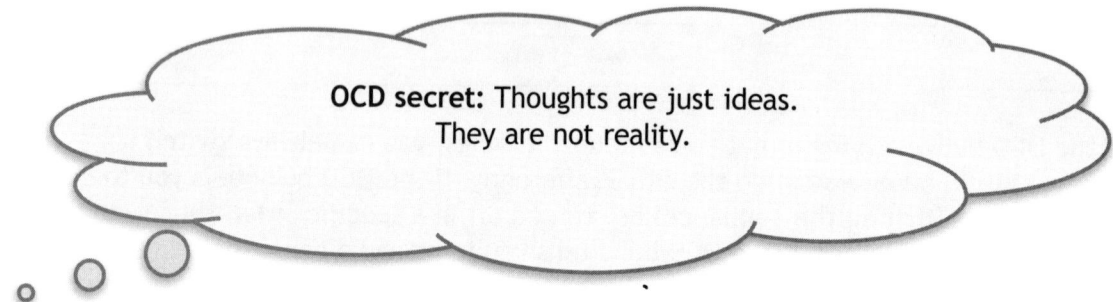

OCD secret: Thoughts are just ideas. They are not reality.

(page 3 of 4)

In-Session ERP Plan

ERP plan: _____

_____

_____

_____

_____

_____

OCD Ruler rating before the ERP: _____

OCD Ruler rating after the ERP: _____

Next steps? _____

_____

_____

_____

_____

_____

_____

_____

_____

_____

_____

From *OCD in Children and Adolescents: The "OCD Is Not the Boss of Me" Manual* by Katherine McKenney, Annie Simpson, and S. Evelyn Stewart. Copyright © 2020 The Guilford Press. Permission to photocopy this material is granted to purchasers of this book for personal use or use with children or youth and their parents (see copyright page for details). Purchasers can download additional copies of this material, in color (see the box at the end of the table of contents).

MODULE 4 HANDOUTS AND WORKSHEETS FOR CHILDREN OR YOUTH

ERP Home Practice for Module 4

ERP task	Goal for the week	Daily homework results
		Day 1:
		Day 2:
		Day 3:
		Day 4:
		Day 5:
		Day 6:
	Reward:	Day 7:
		Day 1:
		Day 2:
		Day 3:
		Day 4:
		Day 5:
		Day 6:
	Reward:	Day 7:
		Day 1:
		Day 2:
		Day 3:
		Day 4:
		Day 5:
		Day 6:
	Reward:	Day 7:

From *OCD in Children and Adolescents: The "OCD Is Not the Boss of Me" Manual* by Katherine McKenney, Annie Simpson, and S. Evelyn Stewart. Copyright © 2020 The Guilford Press. Permission to photocopy this material is granted to purchasers of this book for personal use or use with children or youth and their parents (see copyright page for details). Purchasers can download additional copies of this material, in color (see the box at the end of the table of contents).

MODULE 4 HANDOUTS AND WORKSHEETS FOR PARENTS

Setting Limits on Accommodations

The focus of today's treatment module is on learning how to become on OCD rule breaker. In other words, we focus on identifying ways your child can learn to do the opposite of what OCD wants whenever it pops up. From their experience in the previous weeks, your child has learned that they can break OCD's rules without suffering the feared consequences. There are four ways that your child can break OCD's rules (many of which have been included in your child's weekly ERP homework), and these strategies can be used on a daily basis to show OCD who's boss.

The focus for parents in this module is on addressing family accommodation and how to begin to set limits on OCD-related behaviors. This includes tips on selecting an accommodations to set limits on, discussing limit setting with children, and managing children's reactions to these limits.

Review of Material Covered in the Module 4 Handouts and Worksheets for Children or Youth

The following concepts are presented:

The Four S's: There are four ways in which your child can resist compulsive behaviors in an effort to break OCD's rules. While the goal is always complete resistance, at times children need a more gradual approach. The Four **S**'s include:

- **Shift it:** This strategy involves delaying or postponing a ritual for a specified period of time. In other words, "shift it to later." Delaying a ritual allows for your child's anxiety to increase and then subside without the immediate negative reinforcement offered by the ritual.
- **Shrink it:** This strategy involves reducing the frequency or duration of a ritual. For example, if a child spends 5 minutes washing their hands, then this number can shrink to 4 minutes.
- **Switch it:** This strategy involves completing the ritual in a different manner than that demanded by the OCD. This includes doing the ritual in a different order, location, or time of day; interrupting the ritual with another task; or only completing part of the compulsion.
- **Silly it:** This strategy involves transforming the intrusive thought or compulsive behavior into something ridiculous. This is based on the idea that amusement is a competing response to anxiety and distress. As well, laughing about the OCD thought/ritual makes it less threatening, and therefore easier to resist or boss back. For example, if a child has intrusive thoughts of stabbing a family member, have them imagine using a banana instead.

Limiting Family Accommodation

Parents may want to stop accommodating OCD all at once, despite the fact that doing so would cause significant distress for the child. This desire often stems from a family's fatigue and frustration with having to deal with OCD. Just as your child is gradually moving up their fear hierarchy, you must gradually withdraw accommodations. This means that, at the moment, some accommodation is still necessary, no matter how exhausting it may be.

How to select a target behavior

After completing last week's accommodation monitoring sheet, you should have a better sense about when and how family members may be accommodating your child's OCD. Now it's time to select a target accommodation. The following guidelines can help you make your selection:

1. **It should be a recurrent problem**. The problematic situation should occur relatively frequently in the life of the family so that you can regularly practice setting limits.
2. **It should be something you are motivated to address**. As you begin the process of setting limits on accommodations, your motivation is going to be put to the test, as your child's OCD will push back in reaction to these limits. If you are not highly motivated to address a particular accommodation, you are more likely to abandon your efforts before the goal has been reached.
3. **It should be a significant problem**. The determination of a behavior as "significant" will vary from family to family. Generally, consider behaviors that either impact a child's ability to function in day-to-day life or impact your ability to pursue your own routine and schedule as significant.
4. **It should be something that both you and your child are willing to work on**. Ideally, your child will be in agreement with you about what accommodations to address and how limits will be placed on these behaviors. This agreement will make it easier to manage the expected increases in your child's anxiety when the accommodations are removed or limited. On occasion, a forced choice may be necessary. In other words, parents allow the child to choose between accommodations to target, but choosing none is not an option.

Discussing limit setting

Children and teens may experience a wide variety of reactions to the decision to start limiting accommodations. Some may be pleased that they are receiving some additional support in bossing back the OCD; others may have no initial reaction at all. For some children, the idea of reducing accommodations may triggers feelings of anxiety, distress, or even anger, which can be difficult for parents to tolerate. Regardless of their reactions, it is important for parents to know that in order to win the battle against OCD, parental accommodation must be addressed, with or without the child's approval.

The discussion about limiting accommodations should happen during a time when both you and your child are relaxed. Avoid having this discussion during times when your child's OCD has been triggered and they are demanding your help and reassurance . . . they will be more open to accepting these new limits if they are not anxious.

Here are some other tips to keep in mind during these discussions:

- Acknowledge your child's difficulty in an empathic manner but convey your determination and commitment to overcoming this challenge.
- Focus on **your** intentions, rather than your child's. A discussion that centers around the child (for example, "You can no longer do this") will lead to arguments and noncompliance. In other words, focus on "I" statements, rather than "You" statements.
- If your child reacts in an explosive manner or if previous attempts at talking about this

(page 2 of 4)

subject have been met with difficulties, consider a written announcement. See Leibowitz and Omer's (2013) book for samples of written announcements.

Here is a sample script for how a parent might discuss excessive handwashing and related reassurance-seeking with their child.

> "John, over the past several weeks your mother and I have been learning more about OCD. We know that your fears of getting sick make you really scared and we are really proud of you for trying to face your fears and attend therapy every week. Even though the OCD makes you feel like you need to ask us about handwashing and how clean things are at home when you get these thoughts, we are sure that you will actually be okay even if we don't answer your questions. That's why from now on Mom and Dad are not going to answer your questions when you ask more than once about whether you will get sick. When you manage not to ask us questions more than once, you will earn a reward—a new song on iTunes. If it is too hard for you one day and you ask us questions about illnesses more than once you can always try for the reward again the next day. But even if you do ask, we will not answer after the first time. We know this could be really hard and we are not trying to punish you or hurt you. We love you and want to help you beat the OCD."

This process should be as collaborative as possible, such that the plan is a joint effort by both parents and child to overcome OCD. As much as possible, the child should be included in the planning of the details. In the above example, this may include inviting the child to determine how many questions the parents will initially respond to. When your child agrees to cooperate with limit setting, they should be given as much control as possible over the process in order to reduce conflict and increase "buy in." With that said, parents should refuse to debate with their child the core concept on setting limits on accommodating behaviors.

Examples of limit setting

There are no clear and fast rules about how to set limits on accommodations. The nature of your child's OCD, the type of accommodation in place, and the severity of your child's symptoms will determine how you set limits. Here is a list of ways to set limits for a small sample of accommodations that can help you in your planning.

Participation in washing/cleaning rituals
- parents will not answer questions about their own handwashing
- parents will not allow child to inspect parents hands for cleanliness
- parents will no longer wash clothes more frequently than they do for other members of the household
- parents will not purchase extra cleaning products, soap, or hand sanitizer

Checking behaviors
- parents will not answer questions about whether doors or windows are locked
- parents will not check on their child's behalf
- parents will open doors and windows as they see fit

Avoidance
- parents will not select particular driving or walking routes to avoid triggering the OCD
- parents will not assist with the use of barriers (for example, providing knives and forks to eat finger foods)
- parents will not alter household duties to enable the child to get out of tasks that may trigger anxiety

Even if your child is in agreement with the plan, they are still going to experience an increase in anxiety or distress. It's helpful if parents can be prepared for their child's reaction (as well as their own). This means knowing in advance that your child may feel more anxiety and may be angry at you for this decision.

There are two approaches to managing your child's distress in response to limit setting:

1. **Disengage from your child**. No matter how dramatic or challenging your child's response is to limit setting, remember this: the less you respond, the more quickly it will subside. Parents who can remain disengaged, ignore continued requests for accommodation, and are able to resist becoming drawn into the interaction will quickly see their child become distracted or simply exhausted. In contrast, ongoing discussion will lead to a more drawn-out process. It's as though the OCD is thinking, "As long as we're talking about this, there is a chance that you'll give in!" Disengaging from arguments or provocations is tricky. It may be helpful to role-play with your child not answering them when their anxiety tries to draw you into unproductive discussions.
2. **Distance yourself from your child**. If a child's reactions are aggressive, loud, or explosive, it's best for parents to physically distance themselves from the child until they are calm again (assuming it is safe to do so). Parents should walk away, go to a separate room in the house, or even leave home temporarily rather than respond to the behavior or try to correct it.

Special note: If your child is prone to outbursts, physical aggression, or destruction of property, consider having additional people present in the home when limiting accommodations. The presence of other people besides parents will often inhibit problematic behaviors that a child would otherwise engage in.

With repeated attempts at limit setting, you may notice a change in the way your child reacts to your new approach to dealing with the OCD. At first, a child may become very upset and anxious when you refuse to participate in a ritual. But over time and repeated instances of limit setting, they may become gradually less distressed and recover more quickly. This change reflects your child's ability to cope, as well as a decrease in OCD's strength.

It's important that parents continue to implement reinforcement plans for not only the child's resistance toward OCD (for example, not asking for reassurance, reducing handwashing), but also for having coped with the changes parents have made in terms of accommodations. This does not mean your child must embrace the accommodation; rather, the reinforcement should reflect the fact that they coped with the changes.

For homework this week, use the Limiting Accommodations worksheet on the next page to plan, with your child, what accommodation you'll address and how you will gradually pull back on the behaviors.

MODULE 4 HANDOUTS AND WORKSHEETS FOR PARENTS

Parent Homework for Module 4: Limiting Accommodations

In discussion with your child, select an OCD symptom and related accommodation that the family has implemented that you would like to begin limiting. Together with your child, develop a plan for how to gradually withdraw these behaviors.

OCD symptom	Accommodation	Plan for limit setting

From *OCD in Children and Adolescents: The "OCD Is Not the Boss of Me" Manual* by Katherine McKenney, Annie Simpson, and S. Evelyn Stewart. Copyright © 2020 The Guilford Press. Permission to photocopy this material is granted to purchasers of this book for personal use or use with children or youth and their parents (see copyright page for details). Purchasers can download additional copies of this material, in color (see the box at the end of the table of contents).

MODULE 4 HANDOUTS AND WORKSHEETS FOR PARENTS

Parent Monitoring for Module 4

Each week, monitor the OCD behaviors you observe. These include specific rituals (for example, handwashing, checking), things your child avoids doing, and any OCD-related accommodations that your child requires. Estimate how often these behaviors occur per day and record your response to them (that is, your emotional and/or behavioral reaction). Please bring this sheet with you to the next session.

OCD behaviors (compulsions/avoidance/demands)	Estimated daily average	Parental response

From *OCD in Children and Adolescents: The "OCD Is Not the Boss of Me" Manual* by Katherine McKenney, Annie Simpson, and S. Evelyn Stewart. Copyright © 2020 The Guilford Press. Permission to photocopy this material is granted to purchasers of this book for personal use or use with children or youth and their parents (see copyright page for details). Purchasers can download additional copies of this material, in color (see the box at the end of the table of contents).

MODULE 4 HANDOUTS AND WORKSHEETS FOR PARENTS

Therapist Update for Module 4 (to bring to the next session)

Describe any new symptoms that you noticed over the past week:

_____
_____
_____
_____
_____

Describe any particularly challenging OCD situations that occurred over the week:

_____
_____
_____
_____
_____

Describe any successes that your child experienced over the week:

_____
_____
_____
_____
_____

Is there anything else that you think your child's therapist needs to know about the past week? If so, please describe:

_____
_____
_____
_____
_____

From *OCD in Children and Adolescents: The "OCD Is Not the Boss of Me" Manual* by Katherine McKenney, Annie Simpson, and S. Evelyn Stewart. Copyright © 2020 The Guilford Press. Permission to photocopy this material is granted to purchasers of this book for personal use or use with children or youth and their parents (see copyright page for details). Purchasers can download additional copies of this material, in color (see the box at the end of the table of contents).

MODULE 5

Tools to Help with OCD "Bad Thoughts"
Imaginal Exposures and Dealing with OCD-Related Rage

Imaginal Exposures

Imaginal exposures involve confronting fears in the imagination when it is not feasible or appropriate to confront them in real life. These most often pertain to the "bad thoughts" symptom dimension involving harm-related, sexual, and religious obsessions. Imaginal exposures involve purposefully focusing on distressing thoughts until they become less triggering and provoking.

Worry Scripts

One powerful tool to assist in developing an imaginal exposure is the creation of a worry script. A worry script is a detailed narrative of what the individual fears will happen if they do not perform a related compulsion or avoid the obsessional trigger. A few details to keep in mind when assisting in the creation of a worry script are as follows:

- The worry script should take at least several minutes to read (the longer the better). Three or four sentences will not be enough.
- It should be written in the first person, so words such as "I am . . ." should be used.
- It should be written in the present tense.
- It should be as detailed and vivid as possible, including components such as:
  - Where the individual is when the thought is triggered
  - The content of the anxiety-provoking thoughts and the feared outcome
  - Emotional reactions
  - Rituals that the OCD wants the individual to perform but which are resisted
  - The most catastrophic scenario if the feared outcome came true

The worry script provided below addresses a fear of getting sick from eating expired food. This example may assist you in helping a child or youth develop a worry script specific to their own OCD symptoms.

"I'm sitting at the kitchen table, having just finished my breakfast. I notice a funny aftertaste in my mouth. I faintly detect a sour taste. I run to the fridge and grab the milk carton. As I turn the carton around in my hands, I see the 'best before' date at the bottom. Oh no, the milk expired 3 days ago. I run to the sink to dump out the contents and big curd chunks pour out. But it's too late—I already drank it. My hands are shaking with fear. I can feel the rumbling in my stomach. I bend over from the sharp stabbing cramps. I start to feel clammy and nauseated. I run to the bathroom and kneel in front of the toilet. I can feel the bile start to rise in my throat. I try to swallow it down with deep breaths, but I know it's useless. I rush to pull my hair back just in time for the first wave of vomit. I can feel myself throwing up my undigested breakfast and see it floating in the bowl. Soon, I'm dry heaving as there is nothing left to throw up. After the waves of nausea pass, I'm left sitting on the bathroom floor, feeling weak and disgusting. Now I'll have to miss school today, which means I'll fall behind. And I can't go tomorrow in case I vomit again. I won't be ready for the final exams."

Once the script has been created, it can be used in several ways. The child or youth can begin by setting aside at least 15 minutes each day (the more the better) to repeatedly read over the worry script. The difficulty with reading a worry script is that it is easy for the child or youth to allow their mind to wander, which can detract from the habituation process by avoiding distress induction. However, reading the script can be a good first step if the content is particularly anxiety provoking. Recording and replaying the script on a smartphone is a highly effective and efficient way to promote habituation. The child or youth should record themselves reading the script and then listen to this recording repeatedly for a 15-minute interval every day. When the child or youth makes the recording, it is important that attention be paid to the type of voice and tone they are using. A meek, anxious, quiet voice will convey the message that these words are scary and threatening, whereas a strong, expressive voice will help to promote habituation.

Not surprisingly, children and youth often find the process of creating and reviewing a worry script to be very distressing, and may resist engaging in this activity. Here are some practical pointers to keep in mind:

- If the child or youth appears upset when developing the content of the script, it likely indicates this is an effective worry script. If the child does not seem particularly distressed, this raises the questions of whether the content is specific enough to be triggering and whether the wrong core fear is being targeted. Remember, the creation of the worry script is an exposure in and of itself.

- If the child or youth is not willing to listen to the script, it may be necessary to help them create a new one that is slightly less distress provoking, or to break it up into smaller sections. Once the child has habituated to this less stressful script, they can return to the original version.

- Another way to make a worry script less threatening or distress-provoking is to have the child or youth record while reading it aloud in a funny voice. Options include using an accent, a high-pitched voice, or even a helium-fueled voice. There are also a number of apps that may be of use. For example, Talking Tom or similar apps will repeat what is said in a funny voice. Once children or youth are comfortable with content that is presented in a humorous manner, they can confront the same content in a more distress-provoking format.

Once the child or youth has become bored with the specific narrative, they may need to create a new one that is more vivid and distressing. Another option to maximize usefulness of the script is to have them listen to the worry script when near obsessional triggers. For example, if the script is about contracting HIV, have them listen to it when near a hospital. If the script is about going to hell, have them listen to it while sitting inside a church. They can start with less distress-provoking triggers and then increase the intensity of the triggers as habituation progresses.

CASE EXAMPLE

Sarah is a 13-year-old girl who has been experiencing sexual obsessions related to ego-dystonic doubts about her sexuality. Sarah identifies as heterosexual but has been experiencing intrusive thoughts that she might be attracted to girls. She has been engaging in mental rituals to neutralize this doubt and has been avoiding being in close proximity to girls her age in an effort to prevent triggering her intrusive thoughts. Sarah and her therapist have completed a number of *in vivo* exposures with success, but Sarah continues to be quite distressed by her obsessions. Together Sarah and her therapist have written a detailed worry script, and Sarah has habituated to the content when reading it alone.

> THERAPIST: Sarah, you've done a great job with your worry script over the past week.
>
> SARAH: Thanks. It was really hard when I first started reading it. My distress was like 8 out of 10, but after a while the number went down. Now when I look at this script, I hardly feel anything at all.
>
> THERAPIST: That's wonderful. Now it's time for us to make it more challenging.
>
> SARAH: What does that mean?
>
> THERAPIST: I'd like you to read the script aloud over and over again. Hearing yourself say the words is usually a lot harder than reading the script silently. And it's even harder when someone else is present.
>
> SARAH: This is going to feel so awkward.
>
> THERAPIST: It will at first, but just like you got used to reading the script silently, you'll

get used to reading the script aloud, and then in front of someone. Once you can do that, you can record yourself reading and then listen to the script repeatedly while you're in situations that trigger your obsessions.

SARAH: Like at school?

THERAPIST: Exactly. Listening to the recording while walking in the hallways or riding on the bus would be another way to make the script more challenging. But let's start with reading aloud.

SARAH: My anxiety is already going up.

Making an Appointment with OCD

One way to use imaginal exposures without requiring a worry script is to set aside a specific time for 10 to 20 minutes during the day when the child or youth purposefully focuses on their specific OCD intrusive thoughts in an attempt to habituate to them. This can be done several times per day. This strategy is called *Making an appointment with OCD*. The challenge with this strategy is ensuring that children or youth remain focused on the intrusive thoughts without letting their mind wander to less distressing thoughts. Some approaches to preventing this distraction from happening include ensuring that they are in physical proximity to external obsessional triggers, having obsessions and core fears written down, and not having safety objects nearby. For example, the presence of a parent during this time may make the exposure less triggering. The child or youth may interpret it as being safe to have the thought since the parent will prevent their feared outcome from occurring (e.g., stabbing themselves with a knife). This strategy should not be confused with techniques involving delaying obsessions or "putting worries in a box" to be dealt with at a later time. Delaying obsessions is not a form of exposure and does not enable the child to get used to the intrusive thoughts. But setting aside a time to directly pay attention to the core OCD fears can effectively function as an exposure exercise.

Don't Replace *In Vivo* Exposures with Imaginal Exposures

At times, children and youth may be so resistant to attempting otherwise viable in vivo exposures that it may be tempting to have them imagine themselves performing specific exposures instead. For example, a child who reports being too anxious to touch a contaminated doorknob may ask to instead visualize themselves performing the exposure. However, these types of visualization exercises do little to actually promote habituation and as such run the risk of promoting counterproductive avoidance. It is more effective to develop in vivo exposures that youth will actually attempt, even if they are only minimally distress provoking. As an example, for the child who reports being too anxious to touch a contaminated doorknob, the following options could be presented as alternate initial exposure steps:

- Hover hand close to the doorknob.
- Therapist rubs a tissue on the doorknob and then the child touches the tissue.

- Rub a candy on the doorknob, then the child holds the candy, progressing toward licking and ultimately eating it.
- Rub an article of the child's clothing on the doorknob, then have the child wear it.

Supporting Parents in Managing OCD-Related Rage

In the last module, we discussed helping parents limit family accommodations. This can often result in unexpected coercive or disruptive behavior. Just as different parents will have different experiences in the struggle to limit accommodations, they can have varying degrees of difficulty managing their child's disruptive behavior. Many youth with OCD struggle with OCD-related rage, which can include angry outbursts (e.g., swearing, hurtful comments), destruction of property (e.g., slamming doors, throwing items), and physical aggression toward others (e.g., hitting, kicking, pulling hair). This rage can be in response to a family member not accommodating an OCD-related demand (e.g., when parent enters the child's room without first showering, thereby contaminating a "clean" zone). Youth can also exhibit this behavior out of frustration with how long a ritual is taking, with not being able to get the ritual "right," or because they have been interrupted and need to restart. Some parents report that this is a side of their child they have never seen before, while other parents report that this is a significant worsening of challenging behaviors that their child has always struggled with.

Managing OCD-related rage can be very difficult for parents, and it can be particularly hard for parents to begin to limit accommodations, as outlined in Module 4. A parent handout focused on managing OCD-related rage and aggression is included among the materials at the end of this module. This may be useful to review with all parents, so they are prepared in advance to address OCD-related rage in case it emerges in the future. The handout touches on the following points:

- Respond to disruptive or aggressive behavior in a way that will deescalate the behavior in the moment and reduce the likelihood of future recurrence.
- Violent or aggressive behavior may present as an extreme form of anxiety, reflecting the child's distress rather than personality. In other words, the child or youth is engaging in the "fight" portion of the body's "fight-or-flight" response.
- Prepare for possible outbursts if the child or youth is prone to these types of reactions (identifying triggers, likely locations and behaviors, past parent response and outcomes).
- Instinctive parental responses that escalate disruptive behavior include attempts to negotiate and convince their child, increased parental stress, and impulsive actions.
- Suggest that the parent's goal is to *passively endure* the aggressive or disruptive episode rather than *actively address* it (and get drawn in) in the moment. Respond later once both the child and parent are calm.

It may be helpful for parents to know we have observed that as treatment for OCD progresses, coercive and disruptive behavior decreases (Selles et al., 2018a). Even if you don't directly target this behavior in treatment, it will improve as the OCD symptoms remit.

Homework Assignments

For Module 5, therapists can assign the following for youth and parents to complete at home before the next session.

For Youth

- Practice at least three ERPs daily between sessions. These ERPs are developed in session and recorded on the ERP Home Practice Module 5 worksheet.
- Develop a different worry script (or elaborate on the one created in session) and practice reading it repeatedly for 15 minutes each day. As the child habituates over the week, they can make it more challenging by reading it aloud or recording it and listening to the script repeatedly.

For Parents

- Complete the Parent Monitoring worksheet (parent observations of various compulsions, avoidance behaviors, and accommodations that the child requires, as well as estimated per-day average of each, and how parents responded).
- Complete the Therapist Update worksheet. This worksheet allows parents to share with the child's therapist any new OCD symptoms that were observed over the week, any particularly challenging OCD situations the family encountered, any successes that the child experienced, and any other information parents feel would be helpful for the therapist to know. Therapists should ask parents to provide them with this completed worksheet at the start of the next session so they can address specific issues as needed with the child or with the whole family together.

MODULE 5 HANDOUTS AND WORKSHEETS FOR CHILDREN OR YOUTH

Imaginal Exposures

Over the past modules, you've been working hard on completing ERPs for different compulsions and rituals. Now we're going to learn how to do exposures for the bad thoughts that the OCD bully makes you worry about, like worries about your house burning down, catching a serious illness, or hurting people you care about.

The good news is that we won't put you in situations where these things actually happen. You can learn, however, how to "expose" yourself to the thoughts so they don't cause as much anxiety or distress. This new strategy is called **imaginal exposures.**

Imaginal exposures are just like the exposures you've already been working on except these you'll do with your thoughts instead of behaviors. They include activities like:

- Describe the obsession aloud to your therapist or parent.
- Role-play carrying out the behavior or thought with your therapist.
- Look at pictures of the feared situation or thought.

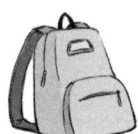

You can also make the exposures a bit silly to help you get through them:

- Sing about the image or idea to the tune of a familiar song.
- Change the image of the feared idea to a silly or ridiculous one.

Just like regular ERPs, you need to do imaginal exposures over and over for a long time in order for you to get used to them. When that happens, these bad thoughts will become background noise that you can ignore.

What kind of imaginal exposure could you do?

_____
_____
_____
_____
_____
_____

(page 1 of 4)

From *OCD in Children and Adolescents: The "OCD Is Not the Boss of Me" Manual* by Katherine McKenney, Annie Simpson, and S. Evelyn Stewart. Copyright © 2020 The Guilford Press. Permission to photocopy this material is granted to purchasers of this book for personal use or use with children or youth and their parents (see copyright page for details). Purchasers can download additional copies of this material, in color (see the box at the end of the table of contents).

One type of imaginal exposure is called a **worry script**. A worry script is a detailed description of your OCD worries, and we use it to bore the OCD bully. Many kids with OCD have a hard time moving past the obsessions and end up spending a lot of time trying to *not* think about the upsetting thoughts. By making a worry script and reading it repeatedly, you get a chance to face these fears directly. The goal is to read the script over and over until the worries no longer bother you. Plan to read the script repeatedly for 15 minutes per day. For example, if the OCD bully made you worry about people in your family being hurt, then the script should include details of the thoughts and images that go along with that obsession. The more detailed, the better!

Here is an example of a worry script about fears of getting sick from eating expired food:

> "Did the milk in my cereal taste a bit funny today? Oh no, maybe it's spoiled. Maybe the date on the milk carton was wrong and it really has expired. I smelled it first but maybe I missed it. I think the milk is sour. I'm going to get sick and throw up. I think my stomach feels a little upset. Yes, I definitely feel sick. Something is wrong with me. I'm definitely nauseous. Oh no, I could have food poisoning. I'm going to throw up all day. Now I'm going to miss school this week and get really behind. I won't pass my test next week. I'm going to fail."

Now it's your turn. Write down your OCD thoughts as they sound to you and try to write them in the order as you experience them. Usually one thought will lead to another. Try not to leave out thoughts because you are afraid of them or because you're worried about the consequences of writing them down.

My Worry Script:

_____

_____

_____

_____

_____

_____

_____

_____

_____

(page 2 of 4)

Another way to use a worry script is to record it and then listen to it out loud over and over. Your parents and therapist can help you figure out how to do this.

Another strategy that can help with bad thoughts is **making an OCD appointment**. Imagine that the OCD bully has you worrying that you might hurt your mother. The first step is to choose a few 10- to 20-minute periods during the day to make an appointment with your OCD bully and take him down! During these times you deliberately invite your thoughts of hurting your mother into your head but don't do any rituals or avoidance behaviors that the OCD bully wants you to do. You're going to purposely repeat the worry over and over as though it were true: *I'm going to hurt my mom. I'm really going to hurt her and she might not survive.* The idea is to stay focused on the thought until your anxiety goes down.

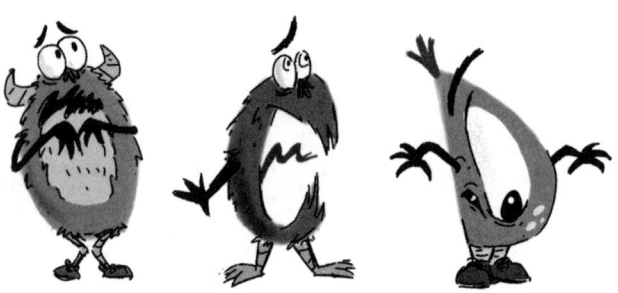

Time for ERPs!

(page 3 of 4)

In-Session ERP Plan

ERP plan: _____

_____

_____

_____

_____

_____

OCD Ruler rating before the ERP: _____

OCD Ruler rating after the ERP: _____

Next steps? _____

_____

_____

_____

_____

_____

_____

_____

_____

_____

_____

_____

MODULE 5 HANDOUTS AND WORKSHEETS FOR CHILDREN OR YOUTH

ERP Home Practice for Module 5

ERP task	Goal for the week	Daily homework results
		Day 1:
		Day 2:
		Day 3:
		Day 4:
		Day 5:
		Day 6:
	Reward:	Day 7:
		Day 1:
		Day 2:
		Day 3:
		Day 4:
		Day 5:
		Day 6:
	Reward:	Day 7:
		Day 1:
		Day 2:
		Day 3:
		Day 4:
		Day 5:
		Day 6:
	Reward:	Day 7:

From *OCD in Children and Adolescents: The "OCD Is Not the Boss of Me" Manual* by Katherine McKenney, Annie Simpson, and S. Evelyn Stewart. Copyright © 2020 The Guilford Press. Permission to photocopy this material is granted to purchasers of this book for personal use or use with children or youth and their parents (see copyright page for details). Purchasers can download additional copies of this material, in color (see the box at the end of the table of contents).

MODULE 5 HANDOUTS AND WORKSHEETS FOR CHILDREN OR YOUTH

Worry Script Practice

Try writing another worry script over the week and read it for 15 minutes each day.

___

Use the chart below to track your practice:

Date	How long did you spend reading over your worry script?	OCD Ruler rating before ERP	OCD Ruler rating after ERP

From *OCD in Children and Adolescents: The "OCD Is Not the Boss of Me" Manual* by Katherine McKenney, Annie Simpson, and S. Evelyn Stewart. Copyright © 2020 The Guilford Press. Permission to photocopy this material is granted to purchasers of this book for personal use or use with children or youth and their parents (see copyright page for details). Purchasers can download additional copies of this material, in color (see the box at the end of the table of contents).

MODULE 5 HANDOUTS AND WORKSHEETS FOR PARENTS

OCD and Rage

The focus of today's module is on imaginal exposures. Imaginal exposures are those that are completed in your child's imagination, rather than *in vivo* (that is, facing fears in real life).

The focus for parents in this module is on managing OCD-related rage and aggression. Rage attacks are relatively common among children and teens with OCD and contribute to family accommodation, which we know can further affect the severity of symptoms and overall impairment. Even if your child has never exhibited this type of behavior, it's important to know how to address OCD-related rage in case it emerges in the future.

Review of Material Covered in the Module 5 Handouts and Worksheets for Children or Youth

Imaginal exposures: When a child fears consequences that cannot be created in real life (for example, burning down the house, a family member dying), the use of imaginal exposures can help the child confront their anxious thoughts. Imaginal exposures (that is, envisioning it in the mind) are based on the same principles as *in vivo* exposures: Extended exposure to obsessional triggers, without ritualizing, will result in habituation and a decreased need to engage in rituals. The difference is that imaginal exposures involve exposing oneself to the thoughts themselves and allowing habituation to the thoughts to occur. There are several ways to conduct imaginal exposures.

- Write down the fears and read them back to yourself.
- Describe the obsession aloud to therapist/parents.
- Listen to a recording of the thought and the feared outcomes.
- Role-play carrying out the behavior or thought with therapist/parent.
- Look at pictures of the feared situation or thought.
- Sing about the image or idea to the tune of a familiar song.
- Change the image of the feared idea to a silly or ridiculous one.

You can also combine imaginal exposures with situational exposures (for example, reading a script of intrusive thoughts regarding burglaries while having left the house without checking that the door is locked). Doing so weakens the bond between obsessions and distress. Imaginal exposures teach the child that obsessional anxiety weakens on its own, and that just thinking about negative events does not mean they will come true.

Worry script: A worry script is a detailed description of your child's OCD worries about a particular topic or obsession that is used to help facilitate habituation to the intrusive thought. Children create a description of their fears and expected negative outcomes that they then read over and over again. Initially, your child's anxiety will be quite high, as they are purposely exposing themselves to the anxiety-provoking thoughts; however, through repeated reading of the script, your child's anxiety in response to the thoughts will begin to decrease. Eventually, they are able to read the scripts with little emotional response. Your child should plan to read the script repeatedly for approximately 15 minutes per day.

(page 1 of 4)

From *OCD in Children and Adolescents: The "OCD Is Not the Boss of Me" Manual* by Katherine McKenney, Annie Simpson, and S. Evelyn Stewart. Copyright © 2020 The Guilford Press. Permission to photocopy this material is granted to purchasers of this book for personal use or use with children or youth and their parents (see copyright page for details). Purchasers can download additional copies of this material, in color (see the box at the end of the table of contents).

Making an OCD appointment: This strategy incorporates the use of imaginal exposures and is particularly good for dealing with intrusive thoughts or mental rituals, such as praying. Making an OCD appointment involves assigning several 10- to 20-minute periods during the day as "worry time" during which the child purposely focuses on the obsession but resists any associated rituals. During the OCD appointment, the child will purposely repeat the obsession over and over as though it was a likely/possible outcome (for example, "I touched the faucet in the public restroom. It's possible I contracted a disease, like HIV"). The challenge is to avoid using any reassurance-type thoughts (for example, "I'll be okay") or other distractions to minimize the anxiety or distress. The goal is for children to make themselves as distressed as they can cope with. With time, the anxiety or distress will subside. The OCD appointment ends when the anxiety or distress is rated as 3 or below on the OCD Ruler.

Dealing with OCD-Related Rage And Aggression

In Module 4, the concepts of disengaging and distancing were introduced. These strategies are key in managing most children's reactions to limiting rituals or accommodations. The focus of this module is to help parents respond to disruptive/aggressive behavior in a way that will deescalate the behavior in the moment and reduce the likelihood of it occurring in the future.

Children with OCD experience a range of emotions when they are triggered by intrusive thoughts, are unable to complete a ritual satisfactorily, or are not accommodated when requested. The emotions include anxiety, frustration, anger, and in some cases, rage and aggression. Families who must cope with these extreme reactions are often baffled as to what to do, since this aggressive behavior is usually out of character for their child and is limited only to OCD-related situations.

OCD-related rage has recently received more attention in the research literature. In the past many children who displayed these types of extreme reactions were misdiagnosed as having oppositional defiant disorder or conduct disorder. We now have a better understanding as to what drives these aggressive responses and how to manage them. It helps for parents to remind themselves that violent or aggressive behavior is most often an extreme form of anxiety, and reflects the child's OCD-related distress rather than their personality. In other words, the child is engaging in the "fight" portion of the "fight-or-flight" response that we learned about in an earlier module.

If you child struggles with OCD-related rage and aggression, you may find Drs. Lebowitz and Omer's SPACE Program (Supportive Parenting for Anxious Childhood Emotions, 2013) to be a helpful resource. We have summarized and adapted several of their strategies here.

If your child is prone to these types of reactions, it is important to prepare yourself for possible outbursts. This involves knowing the following in advance:

- What kind of disruptive/aggressive behavior does the child engage in? Is it physical toward self/others? Is it destructive? Who are the targets?
- What are the triggers for the behavior? This includes various situations, verbal remarks, others' behavior, and so forth.
- Where does the behavior tend to occur?
- How have you as a parent responded in the past and what was the outcome?

(page 2 of 4)

Most people respond to aggressive/disruptive behavior in a way that actually results in more disruptive behavior, rather than less. This is because the child is in a state of heightened arousal that impairs their judgment and perceptions. In this state, parental comments designed to help the situation can be interpreted as combative or threatening. As well, the child's behavior is causing increased parental stress, which can result in parents acting in impulsive ways that can lead to an escalation of the situation.

It's also helpful for parents to shift their understanding of what their goal is in these difficult interactions. Your goal is not to manage the aggressive/disruptive situation; rather, your goal is to endure it while ensuring everyone's safety and resist getting drawn into the interaction (here's where the disengagement skills come in). Your response to the situation will come later when everyone is calm.

1. Delaying Parental Response to Aggressive Behavior

When calm, parents can engage in a sit-in. This technique conveys parental opposition to the aggressive or disruptive behavior and demonstrates parents' commitment to addressing it. The sit-in should only be used in response to serious destructive or aggressive behavior and should be performed no sooner than several hours after the incident. Attempting this strategy immediately following the behavior or while it is occurring will only serve to escalate the conflict. Several hours or even the next day will allow for all parties to be calm and for parents to plan and prepare for the sit-in.

The sit-in involves parents entering the child's room calmly, sitting down, and stating the reason for the meeting (that is, identifying the unacceptable behavior that was exhibited, such as breaking something). Parents state that they will remain in the room and wait for the child to suggest a solution to this problem. Parents can expect to wait between 30 and 60 minutes. The duration depends on the age of the child: younger children require shorter sit-ins. During this time, parents do not engage in conversation with the child or with each other, but will leave if the child offers a solution to the problem. If the child tells parents to leave, parents will remain seated quietly.

If the child offers an acceptable solution (for example, replacing the broken item or going to their room when feeling angry in the future), parents will acknowledge that the idea is reasonable, indicate that they will try that in future, and leave the room. There is no discussion of the sit-in once it is over.

2. Sharing, Not Secrecy

Another strategy that can be helpful in managing aggressive or violent behavior is to inform other people about the details of the child's behavior. The child should be made aware that parents are sharing the details of the behavior with specified people (for example, parents' friends, family members, neighbors) and should be told exactly what information is being shared. Parents can document the disruptive behavior and provide the child with a copy, so there is no misunderstanding of what was shared and with whom. If the child objects, parents can inform the child that violent/aggressive behavior will not be kept a secret and then limit any further discussion on the topic. Knowing that others are aware of their behavior can act as a deterrent for disruptive behavior.

(page 3 of 4)

Those people who are informed of the behavior can also take steps to address the behavior by:

1. Making contact with the child, through e-mail, text, voice mail, or in person.
2. Share their belief in the goodness of the child.
3. Express their specific knowledge of the disruptive behavior.
4. Share their opinion about how aggressive and destructive behavior is unacceptable and how they support the child's parents in their efforts to eliminate the behavior.
5. Express their wish to help the child.

MODULE 5 HANDOUTS AND WORKSHEETS FOR PARENTS

Parent Monitoring for Module 5

Each week, monitor the OCD behaviors you observe. These include specific rituals (for example, handwashing, checking), things your child avoids doing, and any OCD-related accommodations that your child requires. Estimate how often these behaviors occur per day and record your response to them (that is, your emotional and/or behavioral reaction). Please bring this sheet with you to the next session.

OCD behaviors (compulsions/avoidance/demands)	Estimated daily average	Parental response

From *OCD in Children and Adolescents: The "OCD Is Not the Boss of Me" Manual* by Katherine McKenney, Annie Simpson, and S. Evelyn Stewart. Copyright © 2020 The Guilford Press. Permission to photocopy this material is granted to purchasers of this book for personal use or use with children or youth and their parents (see copyright page for details). Purchasers can download additional copies of this material, in color (see the box at the end of the table of contents).

MODULE 5 HANDOUTS AND WORKSHEETS FOR PARENTS

Therapist Update for Module 5 (to bring to the next session)

Describe any new symptoms that you noticed over the past week:

_____
_____
_____
_____
_____

Describe any particularly challenging OCD situations that occurred over the week:

_____
_____
_____
_____
_____

Describe any successes that your child experienced over the week:

_____
_____
_____
_____
_____

Is there anything else that you think your child's therapist needs to know about the past week? If so, please describe:

_____
_____
_____
_____
_____

From *OCD in Children and Adolescents: The "OCD Is Not the Boss of Me" Manual* by Katherine McKenney, Annie Simpson, and S. Evelyn Stewart. Copyright © 2020 The Guilford Press. Permission to photocopy this material is granted to purchasers of this book for personal use or use with children or youth and their parents (see copyright page for details). Purchasers can download additional copies of this material, in color (see the box at the end of the table of contents).

MODULE 6

Tools to Help with ERPs

Coping Cards, Floating On By, Coping with Doubt Scripts, and Reducing Stigma

Coping Cards

This book describes many strategies to teach children and youth about bossing back their OCD. However, not every strategy will work for every individual, so focusing on those techniques that best resonate with a specific child or youth is important for treatment success. One of the strategies that is helpful for almost all children and youth is that of using coping cards. They often experience difficulties in the moment when their OCD is "acting up." To address this, we have them review all of their acquired strategies and boss-back statements and then write some of their favorites on small index cards to keep with them and review during hard situations. Have the child or youth write down different things they can say or do that will help them to get through a sticky obsession without having to avoid a situation or perform a compulsion. Aim to create at least four or five coping cards with the child. It's important that the child or youth does not include any statements that provide reassurance, such as "I'm not going to throw up." or "No one will break into my house." However, statements that reflect the child's ability to cope with the uncertainty regarding negative outcomes are acceptable and helpful, such as "Whatever happens, I know I can cope with it." or "I don't know for sure if the door is locked, but I do know that I'll deal with whatever happens."

The content of coping cards can include different strategies the child has learned, their "boss-back" statements, or anything else that they may find helpful. For example, the child can write things like "A thought is just a thought"; "Just do the opposite of what OCD tells you to do"; or "I don't have to listen to you, OCD. You're not the boss of me!" Children often enjoy decorating their coping cards with stickers and drawings; youth may prefer to store their coping cards as photos on their smartphones for easy access as required.

Floating On By

Teaching the child or youth how to become an observer of their obsessions, rather than a reactor, can be another helpful strategy in managing OCD symptoms. The strategy we call *floating on by* will enable the child to put some distance between themselves and the intrusive thought, which can help to reduce the distress associated with the obsessions and allow the child to more easily resist associated compulsions. This strategy, which is also referred to as cognitive distancing, is borrowed from the ACT literature, and we use the analogies of watching clouds float across the sky, watching fish swim by in an aquarium, and watching trains pass through a station to help children practice observing their thoughts pass by. Just as one does not assign judgments or emotional valences to clouds floating by the sky, we want our clients to allow thoughts to be present without judgments or reactions. Your client can learn to use the following statements when they are bothered by an OCD thought.

- "It's just the OCD bully trying to trick me with these thoughts."
- "These thoughts don't make sense and they're not important."
- "I'm going to keep doing what I'm doing while these thoughts float on by."

Other youth may respond well to incorporating some humor into this approach. Have them greet the OCD thoughts by saying, "Hello OCD thoughts. Welcome. Come on in, there's lots of room. You're allowed to be here. I don't have to do anything about you. I'm going to keep doing what I'm doing while you float on by." Helping clients observe OCD thoughts and teaching them to respond, rather than react, to the obsessions can be a helpful complement to your ERP treatment approach.

Dealing with Doubts

Doubt and uncertainty lie at the core of nearly every obsession, including thoughts such as "How do I know I won't get sick?"; "How can I know for sure that the door is locked?"; "How do I know that I'm straight?"; "Maybe I'm going to hell." It is clear why OCD is referred to as the "doubting disease." OCD doubts demand certainty (or at least the illusion of certainty) through the completion of rituals. Even when the child or youth has been practicing ERPs (*in vivo* and/or imaginal) for several weeks and has made progress with decreasing rituals, doubt and uncertainty often remain. Until these are addressed, there may be a limit on how far treatment gains can progress.

There are several ways in which doubt and uncertainty can be targeted directly in session and in homework:

- Develop worry scripts in which the core fear is the uncertainty itself. The following is a sample worry script regarding doubts about one's sexuality:

"Maybe I am gay, maybe I'm straight. How can I know for sure? Maybe I am attracted to people of the same sex. Maybe I'm bisexual. Maybe I've been fighting my true feelings all my life. Maybe I've been pretending to like boys because that's what all my friends do. Maybe I have actually liked boys. Maybe I'm just discovering my true self now and that's why I'm having all these thoughts. Maybe I'm attracted to both boys and girls, but just didn't know it until now. I'll never know for certain. There's no test for your sexuality. I'll never be 100% certain whether I'm gay, straight, or bisexual."

- If the child or youth engages in excessive reassurance seeking with family members, then coach others to respond in alternative ways that actually expose the child to doubt.

CHILD/YOUTH: Mom, are my hands clean?

MOTHER: That sounds like an OCD question. I don't talk to OCD anymore.

CHILD/YOUTH: Mom, please, just tell me. Are my hands clean?

MOTHER: Maybe they are, maybe they're not. Maybe today is the day you will actually get sick. Maybe it's not. Who knows? I'll guess we'll wait to see what happens.

There are a few things to note about the above example. First, this type of response is best reserved for when parents have already begun the process of setting limits around reassurance. This may include informing the child or youth in advance that this will be the reply. Second, these responses are initially very frustrating for children, and parents should be prepared for initial worsening of reassurance-seeking behaviors before they remit. Third, these responses not only limit parental accommodations by refusing to give the OCD its desired response, but they also serve to expose the child or youth to the underlying doubt with which they are struggling to cope.

- In-session exposures may also include a discussion with the child about the underlying OCD-driven doubt. Below is an example designed to target a child's uncertainty whether they will contract HIV from touching household items.

CHILD/YOUTH: I might get HIV from drinking from this cup. Who knows? I'll never know how big a risk I'm at.

THERAPIST: That's right. Who knows? Maybe someone with HIV also drank from that same cup before you. Maybe they had an open sore in their mouth, and a minute amount of their blood got into the cup. Maybe you've just been exposed to HIV-infected blood. Maybe you've contracted the virus.

CHILD/YOUTH: Maybe. Maybe the virus is spreading throughout my bloodstream as we speak. Maybe my immune system is already compromised.

THERAPIST: Maybe. We'll never know if you put yourself at risk. Maybe you did, maybe you didn't. Maybe you're HIV positive, maybe you're not.

- Engaging in this type of exposure for 5 to 10 minutes will lead to habituation to the thoughts, as well as a growing realization of the irrationality of living in constant fear of contracting HIV.

Coping with Doubt Scripts

When a child or youth is participating in an *in vivo* exposure (either at home or in session), the use of a coping script can be very useful in helping them to ride out their distress while resisting rituals. Coping with doubt scripts (as the name implies) help an individual cope with OCD-driven uncertainty. The scripts are best viewed as temporary measures to help a child or youth get through a difficult planned ERP (or an unexpected trigger that is encountered during the day) when the urge to do a ritual becomes very strong. The risk of relying on a coping script for every exposure (either planned or spontaneous) is that reading the script may become a ritual in and of itself. This potential should be monitored in sessions. Some youth prefer to type the script into their phones so that they have a less intrusive means of accessing it when needed. An example of a coping with doubt script follows:

> "I can never know for sure that I locked the front door. Even if I go back and check, or replay the scene in my head 100 times, I cannot be 100% certain. Even if I checked, it's possible that the lock is faulty or that the lock did not fully close. Checking won't accomplish anything and will make my OCD worse. If I am going to have a better life, I must fight the OCD bully and resist the urge to check. I must be okay with knowing it is possible that the door is unlocked. I know that the OCD bully has made life hard for me and it will keep getting worse if I keep checking. I have made a commitment to do the opposite of what the OCD bully wants me to do so I will resist the urge to go back and check the door."

Components of a Coping with Doubt Script

There are several components of a coping with doubt script, including acknowledging the doubt and inability to obtain 100% certainty; stating a commitment to overcoming OCD;, and recognizing one's ability to cope with whatever happens as an outcome. When developing a coping with doubt script with a child or youth, it is often helpful to use the above example as a template and modify the content to fit their specific symptoms. It is very important that the coping with doubt script not include subtle messages of reassurance that will interfere with the habituation process.

CASE EXAMPLE

Jane is a 16-year-old girl who has struggled with OCD since age 10. She experiences harm-related obsessions and worries that she will be responsible for something bad happening to her home. She repeatedly checks to make sure appliances and other electrical items are unplugged before leaving the house and before going to bed. Jane worries a lot of about house fires and fears that by leaving something plugged in, she could cause her house to burn down. She is struggling in treatment to resist checking as part of her ERPs.

THERAPIST: Jane, you've been doing a great job at trying the ERPs that we plan in session, but it still seems that it's really hard for you to resist the urge to check things like your hair straightener and the lamps before bed.

JANE: I'm trying, okay? I've been able to delay checking for 10 minutes.

THERAPIST: I know. You're really pushing yourself and it's not easy. I think it might help if we work on a coping with doubt script that you can use when you're at home and trying not to check at night.

JANE: I don't get it.

THERAPIST: A coping with doubt script is something you can read when you're unexpectedly triggered and you're trying to resist your compulsions. A coping with doubt script reminds you that there are no guarantees and no certainty in life, even if OCD wants you to believe otherwise. And that it you want a life free from OCD then you have to be willing to tolerate that uncertainty without doing your rituals.

JANE: That sounds horrible.

THERAPIST: (*Chuckles.*) Let's give it a try and then see what you think.

OCD Disclosure and Reducing Stigma

Many children, youth, and families live under a veil of secrecy when it comes to the diagnosis of OCD. Unfortunately, notable stigma persists around mental illness in general, which limits parents' comfort with disclosing their child's struggle with OCD. There is also a fundamental misunderstanding among the general public related to OCD and its impairment. The casual phrase "I'm so OCD about that" is heard regularly and detracts from awareness of the true debilitating and impairing nature of OCD.

One way that families can reduce the stigma of OCD is to start the process of disclosing information about their child's struggle with OCD and how treatment has positively impacted their lives. Disclosing this kind of information to trusted individuals can go a long way in helping a child or youth to feel empowered and to feel as though they are taking control back from OCD. OCD thrives off of secrecy, so the more open a child or youth is about their symptoms, the less power OCD tends to have over their life. The decision to share this personal information should be made collaboratively, and the child or youth should be involved in deciding who to share this information with, what information is shared, and how the information is shared. Some children or youth prefer to speak with specific individuals face to face, while others may prefer to describe their OCD and treatment progress in a letter, text, or e-mail. Children usually experience a tremendous sense of relief and pride in being able to talk about their struggle with OCD, as well as how treatment has positively impacted their lives, as those they speak with almost always respond with empathy, support, and encouragement. Over the years, we have received proud reports from families after their child gave a classroom presentation on OCD or completed a project on this topic.

Homework Assignments

For Module 6, therapists can assign the following for youth and parents to complete at home before the next session:

For Youth

Practice at least three ERPs daily between sessions. These ERPs are developed in session and recorded on the ERP Home Practice for Module 5 worksheet.

For Parents

- Complete the Parent Monitoring worksheet (parent observations of various compulsions, avoidance behaviors, and accommodations that the child requires, as well as estimated per-day average of each, and how parents responded).
- Complete the Therapist Update worksheet. This worksheet allows parents to share with the child's therapist any new OCD symptoms that were observed over the week, any particularly challenging OCD situations the family encountered, any successes that the child experienced, and any other information parents feel would be helpful for the therapist to know. Therapists should ask parents to provide them with this completed sheet at the start of the next session so they can address specific issues as needed with the child or with the whole family together.

MODULE 6 HANDOUTS AND WORKSHEETS FOR CHILDREN OR YOUTH

Tools to Help with ERPs

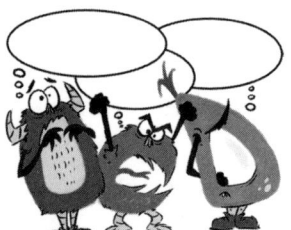

Another way the OCD bully can cause problems for you is through doubt . . . doubting whether you locked the door, doubting whether your schoolwork is good enough, doubting whether you made a mistake. That's why OCD is often referred to as "the doubting disease." To manage these feelings of doubt, OCD makes you check or do other things to make sure. The OCD bully likes things to be 100% certain. Hopefully this program has taught you that there's no such thing! Nothing in life is 100% certain.

In other words:

You have to learn to live with a certain amount of uncertainty

One strategy that can be really helpful in coping with doubt is to develop a **coping with doubt script.** The purpose of a coping with doubt script is to help you manage those situations where doubt or anxious thoughts make it difficult for you to resist compulsions or to face your anxious triggers. Here's an example of a coping with doubt script for dealing with doubts about locking a door:

> "I can never know for sure that I locked the front door. Even if I go back and check, or replay the scene in my head 100 times, I cannot be 100% certain. Even if I checked, it's possible that the lock is faulty or that the lock did not fully close. Checking won't accomplish anything and will make my OCD worse. If I am going to have a better life, I must fight the OCD bully and resist the urge to check. I must be okay knowing it is possible that the door is unlocked. I know the OCD bully has made life hard for me and it will keep getting worse if I keep checking. If I do find out the front door was unlocked and someone broke in, I will deal with it and get on with my life. Bad things happen and people find ways to cope. I have made a commitment to do the opposite of what the OCD bully wants me to do, so I will resist the urge to go back and check the door."

A coping with doubt script is not about getting reassurance for your obsession, it's about helping you manage anxious thoughts, resist compulsions, and confirm your commitment to no longer give in to the OCD bully's demands. It's also not meant to be used forever or as part of a ritual. It's a temporary strategy to help you cope during tough ERPs or when you are unexpectedly faced with an OCD trigger and need help to ride out the urge to do a compulsion.

Now it's your turn to write a coping with doubt script for one of your obsessions:

My obsession: _____

My compulsion/ritual/avoidance behavior: _____
_____
_____

My coping with doubt script: _____
_____
_____
_____
_____
_____
_____
_____
_____
_____
_____
_____
_____
_____

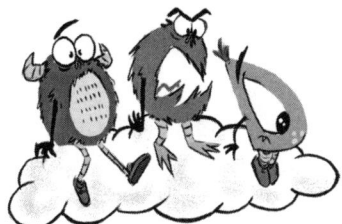

If you think about obsessions for a moment, you'll realize that they come and go. They're not present in every situation and they're not present all the time. Obsessions float in when they want to, like the wind and the clouds in the sky. You don't do anything to make them happen; they have a mind of their own. Sometimes obsessions show up in response to triggers and sometimes they just show up. Obsessions also pass by on their own.

When an obsession just shows up, treat it like a cloud passing in the sky, birds flying overhead, fish swimming past in an aquarium, or a train passing through a station. These objects, just like obsessive thoughts, are neither good nor bad . . . they're just there. Try to avoid judgments about these thoughts and what they mean about you. Rather, just watch them come and then watch them go.

(page 2 of 5)

Here's how you do this: When an obsession pops into your head, you need to see it, recognize what it is, label it as unimportant, and continue with what you were doing. The point of letting obsessions pass through is that the OCD bully gets stronger when it gets a reaction out of you. When you allow the obsessions to come and go without reacting to them, they tend to weaken naturally.

When you let obsessions come and go without reacting, you're using a strategy called **floating on by**. The OCD bully will go away because the things that feed it, like avoidance, intense feelings, and rituals, aren't present. With this strategy, you're not trying to challenge the obsession—you're trying to change how you react to it.

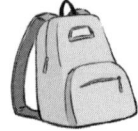

Here are three statements that you can use when the OCD bully makes an appearance:

1. It's just the OCD bully trying to trick me with these thoughts.
2. These thoughts don't make sense and they're not important.
3. I'm going to keep doing what I'm doing while these thoughts float on by.

If you're able to boss back the OCD bully, then go right ahead. The strategy of allowing the OCD thoughts to float on by is a good one to use when bossing back a particular obsession isn't working that well and you find yourself getting more and more upset. Take a deep breath and allow the thoughts to go floating on by.

By now, your backpack is getting pretty heavy with all the different strategies you've learned. But we need to make room for one more!

When the OCD bully is at its sneakiest, it can be really hard to think back on all the strategies you've learned and the different ways to boss it back. It would be great if you could take all these papers with you wherever you went so you could review your strategies whenever the OCD bully starts to cause problems. Having your treatment materials with you all the time is pretty silly. Plus, most kids feel a little embarrassed about looking through their papers with other people around.

So today we're going to squeeze all the important information in these papers onto small pieces of paper called **coping cards**. Coping cards are small reminders that you can keep with you at all times that will help you out in hard OCD situations. We're going to write down different things you can do or say that will help you get through a tough obsession without having to avoid something or do a compulsion.

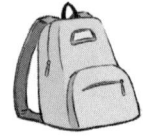

Write down all the things you would like on your coping cards. You can write the different strategies you've learned, ways to boss back the OCD bully, secrets the OCD bully doesn't want you to know, or just about anything else you would find helpful. These can fit in your pocket or you can take a picture of them with a phone.

(page 3 of 5)

1. _____
2. _____
3. _____
4. _____
5. _____
6. _____
7. _____
8. _____
9. _____
10. _____

Time for more practice . . .

In-Session ERP Plan

ERP plan: _____

_____

_____

_____

_____

_____

OCD Ruler rating before the ERP: _____

OCD Ruler rating after the ERP: _____

Next steps? _____

_____

_____

_____

_____

_____

_____

_____

_____

_____

_____

From *OCD in Children and Adolescents: The "OCD Is Not the Boss of Me" Manual* by Katherine McKenney, Annie Simpson, and S. Evelyn Stewart. Copyright © 2020 The Guilford Press. Permission to photocopy this material is granted to purchasers of this book for personal use or use with children or youth and their parents (see copyright page for details). Purchasers can download additional copies of this material, in color (see the box at the end of the table of contents).

MODULE 6 HANDOUTS AND WORKSHEETS FOR CHILDREN OR YOUTH

ERP Home Practice for Module 6

ERP task	Goal for the week	Daily homework results
		Day 1:
		Day 2:
		Day 3:
		Day 4:
		Day 5:
		Day 6:
	Reward:	Day 7:
		Day 1:
		Day 2:
		Day 3:
		Day 4:
		Day 5:
		Day 6:
	Reward:	Day 7:
		Day 1:
		Day 2:
		Day 3:
		Day 4:
		Day 5:
		Day 6:
	Reward:	Day 7:

From *OCD in Children and Adolescents: The "OCD Is Not the Boss of Me" Manual* by Katherine McKenney, Annie Simpson, and S. Evelyn Stewart. Copyright © 2020 The Guilford Press. Permission to photocopy this material is granted to purchasers of this book for personal use or use with children or youth and their parents (see copyright page for details). Purchasers can download additional copies of this material, in color (see the box at the end of the table of contents).

MODULE 6 HANDOUTS AND WORKSHEETS FOR PARENTS

Destigmatizing OCD

The focus of today's treatment session is on learning three additional strategies that can help children be successful with their ERPs: (1) coping with doubt script, (2) floating on by, which is a form of cognitive detachment, and (3) coping cards, which are reminders of strategies, OCD secrets, and ways to boss back the OCD that your child can keep with them to use during difficult OCD situations.

The focus for parents in this module is on managing stigma associated with OCD. Parents and children often have a number of concerns about the impact of others knowing about the OCD, and they struggle with who and what to tell. While a more open approach can be helpful in treatment, there can be repercussions to disclosing too much information.

Review of Material Covered in the Module 6 Handouts and Worksheets for Children or Youth

The following concepts are presented:

Coping with doubt script: OCD is often referred to as the "doubting disease" . . . doubting whether you locked the door, doubting whether your hands are clean enough, doubting whether you made a mistake. To alleviate these uncomfortable feelings of doubt, OCD requires your child to check, repeat activities, or do other tasks to make sure. The problem? Nothing in life is 100% certain. One strategy that can be helpful in dealing with doubt is the use of coping with doubt scripts, which are designed to help children manage the distress associated with uncertainty. Here is an example of a coping with doubt script for addressing doubts about whether a door is locked:

> "I can never know for sure that I locked the front door. Even if I go back and check, or replay the scene in my head 100 times, I cannot be 100% certain. Even if I checked, it's possible that the lock is faulty or that the lock did not fully engage. Checking won't accomplish anything and will make my OCD worse. If I am going to have a better life, I must fight my OCD and resist the urge to check. I must go on knowing it is possible that the door is unlocked. I know the OCD has made life hard for me and it will keep getting worse if I keep checking. If I do find out the front door was unlocked and someone broke in, I will deal with it and get on with my life. Bad things happen and people find ways to cope. I have made a commitment to do the opposite of what OCD wants me to do, so I will resist the urge to go back and check the door."

A coping with doubt script is not about your child obtaining reassurance for their fears. Rather, coping with doubt scripts are designed to help your child manage the distressing thought, resist the compulsion, and confirm their commitment to no longer give in to OCD's demands. Coping with doubt scripts are not meant to be used indefinitely, nor are they meant to be used ritualistically. A coping with doubt script is a temporary strategy to help your child cope with

(page 1 of 3)

From *OCD in Children and Adolescents: The "OCD Is Not the Boss of Me" Manual* by Katherine McKenney, Annie Simpson, and S. Evelyn Stewart. Copyright © 2020 The Guilford Press. Permission to photocopy this material is granted to purchasers of this book for personal use or use with children or youth and their parents (see copyright page for details). Purchasers can download additional copies of this material, in color (see the box at the end of the table of contents).

ERPs and anxious triggers until habituation has occurred. In session, your child will be asked to develop a coping with doubt script for their own OCD fear.

Floating on by: Before treatment, your child had strong reactions to their intrusive thoughts . . . they likely thought it meant something about them, that they had to do a ritual to get rid of them, or use other techniques to get rid of the thoughts (for example, distraction, pushing them away). This program has taught your child to react differently to these thoughts by bossing them back and challenging the logic of what OCD wants them to believe. **Floating on by** is another cognitive strategy your child can use and is probably one of the most effective, albeit challenging, tools to put into practice. This strategy, which is a form of cognitive detachment, helps the child to distance themselves and disengage attention from the upsetting intrusive thoughts that characterize OCD. We ask children to see OCD as though it were a cloud passing in the sky, birds flying overhead, fish swimming past in an aquarium, or a train passing through a station. Like OCD, all of these things appear and then pass by without any necessary intervention, except recognizing that they are present only for a limited time. **Floating on by** involves teaching your child three statements that they can use when bothered by an OCD thought:

1. **It's just the OCD bully trying to trick me with these thoughts** (this allows the child to recognize the thought as belonging to OCD and not their own thought or an idea that means something about themselves)
2. **These thoughts don't make sense and they're not important** (this implies that the OCD thought is nonsensical and meaningless, therefore no response is necessary)
3. **I'm going to keep doing what I'm doing while these thoughts float on by** (this highlights the fact that the symptom will pass on its own if nothing is done)

None of these statements includes any judgments about the thoughts, nor do they imply that one must avoid obsessive triggers or perform a ritual.

Coping cards: When struggling with a difficult ERP, or encountering a distress-provoking trigger out of the blue, it can be challenging to remember all the different strategies or ways to boss back the OCD that your child has learned in session. It can be helpful to have reminders written on 3" × 5" cards that can be kept on hand and referred to when needed. In other words, coping cards are like an OCD cheat sheet. In session, we will be generating a list of helpful statements your child can use that will include a combination of bossing-back statements, cognitive restructuring, and facilitating detachment, as well as OCD secrets and other strategies.

Destigmatizing OCD

Despite the fact that there has been great progress made in destigmatizing mental illness over the last 10 to 20 years we still have a way to go before we see it in the same way as we see most physical illness. Media coverage and portrayals of OCD in movies and on television tend to rely on sensational depictions or stereotypes, rather than facts, which can impact the perception of the disorder and reinforce the stigma of mental illness.

(page 2 of 3)

Stigma can be experienced in different ways, including obvious and direct forms (for example, a peer making a negative comment about the OCD or treatment) or subtle ways (for example, peers assume child is unstable or "crazy" because of the OCD). Regardless of the form, stigma is one of the reasons why it takes an average of 14–17 years from the time of symptom onset for people to access treatment for OCD. One of the biggest barriers for children and families accessing treatment is the stigma and potential discrimination associated with OCD. And those who do obtain treatment often keep this therapy a secret.

For many of you, as parents, the stigma you and your child may face may be one of the biggest concerns you have for your child. You may have asked yourself questions such as:

- "How will teachers and my child's peers treat them if they find out about the OCD?"
- "What about my child's employment options?"
- "How will my child manage school demands?"
- "How can my child manage romantic relationships?"

How much and who to tell (about the OCD) are questions that many parents struggle with. On the one hand we know that being more open about the OCD is generally the better approach to managing it, as OCD thrives on secrecy. On the other hand, we do not want our children to be faced with possible repercussions from having shared their struggles with OCD. There are no set rules around what course to take, but likely it is best to proceed with some caution, allowing time and your and your child's comfort level to guide you.

Sooner or later it makes sense to let those people closer to your family know about the OCD. Often these people will have some idea that there is a problem already. Talking to teachers, friends, and family members about OCD and its effects, and how you would like them to handle this knowledge may well be a relief for everyone. Of course it is best if you and your child are on the same page as to the who, when, and where of it. This may take some working out.

For people less close to your child/family it may be less wise to be completely open about the details of your child's OCD, particularly if you feel it may negatively impact your child in some way. Your child will be developing their own approach to sharing information and you may need to respect their pacing for divulging information.

If your family decides to disclose your child's OCD to people outside your family, it's important to consider the manner in which this information is shared. We live in the world of text messages, social networking sites, blogs, e-mail, and YouTube. While these forms of communication are now an important way in which we connect with others, particularly for young people, they are also permanent. And we often cannot control how that information is shared, with whom, and for how long once it is posted online. So if and when your child is ready to share their struggles with OCD with others, it may be best to do it face-to-face.

MODULE 6 HANDOUTS AND WORKSHEETS FOR PARENTS

Parent Monitoring for Module 6

Each week, monitor the OCD behaviors you observe. These include specific rituals (for example, handwashing, checking), things your child avoids doing, and any OCD-related accommodations that your child requires. Estimate how often these behaviors occur per day and record your response to them (that is, your emotional and/or behavioral reaction). Please bring this sheet with you to the next session.

OCD behaviors (compulsions/avoidance/demands)	Estimated daily average	Parental response

From *OCD in Children and Adolescents: The "OCD Is Not the Boss of Me" Manual* by Katherine McKenney, Annie Simpson, and S. Evelyn Stewart. Copyright © 2020 The Guilford Press. Permission to photocopy this material is granted to purchasers of this book for personal use or use with children or youth and their parents (see copyright page for details). Purchasers can download additional copies of this material, in color (see the box at the end of the table of contents).

MODULE 6 HANDOUTS AND WORKSHEETS FOR PARENTS

Therapist Update for Module 6 (to bring to the next session)

Describe any new symptoms that you noticed over the past week:

_____
_____
_____
_____
_____
_____

Describe any particularly challenging OCD situations that occurred over the week:

_____
_____
_____
_____
_____
_____

Describe any successes that your child experienced over the week:

_____
_____
_____
_____
_____
_____

Is there anything else that you think your child's therapist needs to know about the past week? If so, please describe:

_____
_____
_____
_____
_____

From OCD in Children and Adolescents: The "OCD Is Not the Boss of Me" Manual by Katherine McKenney, Annie Simpson, and S. Evelyn Stewart. Copyright © 2020 The Guilford Press. Permission to photocopy this material is granted to purchasers of this book for personal use or use with children or youth and their parents (see copyright page for details). Purchasers can download additional copies of this material, in color (see the box at the end of the table of contents).

MODULE 7

Troubleshooting ERPs

Suboptimal Response, Therapist Pitfalls, and Barriers to Treatment Success

The treatment materials in Module 7 are focused on encouraging the child to take risks in their ERPs. This may involve attempting ERPs that were listed near the top of their OCD Ladder, combining imaginal exposures with very distress-provoking obsessional triggers, or even engaging in exposures that may at one time have seemed unimaginable. Having the child first visualize themselves attempting and then successfully completing an ERP can prime them for actually attempting the same exposure, much like a professional baseball player might visualize hitting a home run before stepping up to the plate. This use of visualization should not be considered a form of imaginal exposure, as we are not asking the child to imagine themselves touching a doorknob, for example. Rather, we are asking the child to visualize touching the doorknob, imagine experiencing the expected increase in distress, and then imagine that distress decreasing over time as they ride out the urge to engage in a washing compulsion. We then ask the child to follow this visualization activity with the same ERP in real life. Therapists can support this activity by providing the step-by-step description of the ERP that is being visualized, including the increase and subsequent decrease in distress.

At this point in the treatment process, you have likely experienced many successes with children and their parents; however, if you're like most therapists who treat OCD, you've probably also encountered challenges with various ERPs. It may be that an ERP you have developed is not distressing enough, or perhaps too distressing, resulting in the youth bailing out of the exposure too soon. Perhaps an ERP conducted in the office was successful, but the same activity at home was a disaster. Or perhaps the child's anxiety and/or distress does not seem to decrease over time. There are several factors that a therapist should explore if ERPs do not seem to be going as planned, as outlined below.

What If ERPs Are Not Working?

Imagine the following scenario: You have developed what seems like the perfect ERP. You are confident that you know what the child or youth's OCD-related core fear is, you have identified the obsessional triggers (both internal and external), and you have targeted compulsions thus far in a gradual fashion. You are certain that you have crafted an effective ERP that is creative and engaging. What could possibly go wrong? In actuality, a multitude of factors could interfere with achieving a good response. If an ERP is not evoking the desired level of distress, consider the following possible explanations:

- The child or youth may be avoiding strong emotions by using subtle distraction (directing their thoughts to other topics) or by dulling themselves to the distress. They could be saying to themselves, "I'm doing this because my therapist told me to" or "It's not really me who's doing this." Therapists should check in during the exposure to determine what the child or youth is thinking to keep them engaged with the distress-provoking material.

- The presence of other people during exposures can serve as a subtle safety signal at times. This person could be a parent who repeatedly reminds their child that they are safe and that nothing bad will happen to them because of the ERP. These safety signals can also be much more covert. The presence of a therapist can also signal safety if the child or youth believes that a therapist would never allow them to do something dangerous. Similarly, they may interpret a therapist's lack of response to reassurance seeking as confirmation that everything will be okay. In these instances, it is important for therapists to introduce doubt into the safety of the ERP, as demonstrated in the following interaction:

    THERAPIST: Great job touching the raw meat.

    CHILD: Are you sure it's not contaminated with *E. coli*? What if I get sick?

    THERAPIST: Sorry, buddy. I'm not a microbiologist. There is no way for us to know if the meat is contaminated. I don't know if you'll get sick, but I do know we'll get through whatever happens.

These statements inducing doubt are often experienced as distressing by children and youth with OCD, and are best introduced gradually.

- At times, children and youth will willingly and easily complete an exposure that should be quite challenging for them. The problem may not be with the exposure itself, but rather that children tell themselves they will undo or neutralize the anxiety or negative feelings with a ritual at a later time (e.g., after the session, as a part of their washing routine). In these instances, it is important to be explicit about how long the child has to wait before engaging in a ritual. This delay should be long enough to allow the child's distress to decrease noticeably. The child may be willing to delay the ritual even longer if bonus rewards are introduced. For example, the child can earn an extra minute of screen time for every additional minute that they delay the ritual.

- During particularly distress-provoking ERPs, children and youth may find that they are distancing themselves from the experience, such that they tell themselves, "It's not me doing this ERP." At a more extreme level, children and youth may dissociate during the experience. This can be managed by helping to ground the child (e.g., light touch on the shoulder that you've agreed upon in advance) in the moment, checking in on their distress level, and using other strategies to ensure that they remain present in the moment.

- Another possibility is that the child or youth has replaced the targeted compulsion with another ritual, thereby undoing the effectiveness of the ERP. This is particularly tricky to uncover if a physical compulsion has been replaced with a mental ritual. For example, a child or youth may be able to easily resist handwashing rituals if they are repeating prayers in their head that provide reassurance (e.g., "Dear God, please keep me healthy and clean"). It is helpful to periodically check with the child on whether they are doing any mental rituals to alleviate their distress.

- An exposure may not be triggering distress because the child or youth, or family members, has taken steps to ensure that the feared act will not occur. For example, a common accommodation in families in which the child or youth has fears of stabbing a family member is to remove all the knives and sharp objects from the home. Similarly, if a child or youth is worried that they could be poisoned by household cleaners, family members may have already replaced toxic cleaners with nontoxic cleaning products. These safety behaviors will inherently lower a child or youth's distress during imaginal exposures, since precautions have already been taken to prevent the feared outcome. Therapists should check with the child or youth and parents on whether any safety measures have already been implemented. If so, these should be removed in a stepwise fashion.

- Children and youth can be excessively perfectionistic in how they carry out exposures, which can interfere with the effectiveness of the ERP. For example, they may be excessively monitoring their distress to ensure that it is at the targeted level, which results in distraction and a lack of habituation. Similarly, a child or youth who strives to execute the "perfect" ERP may never actually get started. Or if a child or youth feels that the ERP is not going perfectly, they may discontinue the exposure before habituation has occurred. This can be addressed by targeting perfectionism directly in exposures (e.g., making mistakes on purpose).

Therapist Pitfalls

Treating OCD can be a tricky process. OCD treatment is full of pitfalls for novice (and not-so-novice) therapists. In this section, we discuss a list of 10 common therapist pitfalls with suggestions on how to avoid and address them.

Pitfall 1: Inadvertently Providing Reassurance

OCD is sneaky! It works very hard to get what it wants; and often what it wants is reassurance that the feared outcome will not occur. As presented earlier, OCD often gets children and youth to ask many, many, many questions of trusted adults. It is important to remember that one of these trusted adults is the therapist. Reassurance seeking is a core feature in OCD. By obtaining answers to questions, children and youth receive the message that they are unable to tolerate the discomfort associated with uncertainty.

It is easy enough for therapists to refrain from making statements such as "You are going to be okay"; "You are not going to get sick"; or "You are not going to hurt someone." However, there are sneakier ways that OCD will try to get children to gain reassurance for which you must be on the lookout. For example, the child or youth may comment, "I'm probably not going to get sick, right?" Responding with "yes," or even saying nothing at all, can be taken as confirmation that the child or youth will be okay. At times, even the simple presence of a therapist can be experienced as reassurance; a child or youth will think, "Well, my therapist wouldn't actually put me in harm's way."

So, what is a therapist to do when OCD is this sneaky? If you begin to suspect that the child or youth is gaining reassurance either overtly or covertly, be sure to introduce doubt and uncertainty into the exposures. Again, the goal is for the child or youth to learn how to tolerate uncertainty, as it is certainty that OCD is demanding! Introducing ideas such as "You may get sick; you might not. There is no way of knowing," or saying things like "Maybe yes, maybe no" will inject doubt into the exposures, preventing the therapist from succumbing to this pitfall.

Pitfall 2: Answering Questions about Uncertainty

A related pitfall is answering questions about uncertainty itself. For example, therapists can often get caught up in discussions with children about whether a symptom is really OCD and how this is really known. Children or youth might ask, "How do you know this is OCD and I'm not a bad person who really does want to kill my mom?," and so forth. The therapist can easily be drawn into providing evidence to support why a symptom is consistent with OCD and providing disproving evidence that suggests otherwise. When a child recurrently asks questions about whether a thought is OCD or not, this is likely an attempt to achieve certainty, such that answering those questions removes momentary distress, providing reinforcement and increasing the likelihood of future questions.

Similar to the situation described in Pitfall 1, introducing the element of doubt and uncertainty is key. You can say something like the following: "I can never know for certain that it is OCD and it *is* possible that you might go and kill your mother when you get home." In this way, the therapist helps the child or youth learn to tolerate this doubt. At the very least, it decreases the chances that the child will ask the question again, since it did not achieve OCD's goal of gaining certainty.

Pitfall 3: Moving Too Fast Up the OCD Ladder

Another pitfall that sometimes occurs is inadvertently moving too fast up the OCD ladder. Often children and youth just want to "white-knuckle it" and move as quickly as possible up the OCD ladder, without giving themselves a chance to habituate to the distress connected with lower steps. The key is for the child or youth to experience the distress decreasing naturally without having to engage in a ritual. When children or youth race up the ladder, just to check off challenges on the list, they don't allow themselves to experience habituation. Therefore, each step needs to be completed for long enough and frequently enough to promote lasting change. Similarity, if the clinician starts a task that is too high up the ladder and the ERP is too distress provoking, the child or youth may not be successful and may resort to escaping the situation by doing a ritual, thereby reinforcing the OCD. This can contribute to a child or youth's sense a failure and helplessness, thereby decreasing motivation and engagement in therapy.

Pitfall 4: Moving Too Slowly or Spending Too Much Time Discussing the OCD Ladder

The opposite of Pitfall 3 can occur as well, when the therapist is afraid to push the child or youth. While it can be very challenging to tolerate the distress of the child or youth, it is crucial to not underestimate their capacity to succeed. If therapy proceeds too slowly, this limits progress by denying the child or youth the opportunity to build momentum and experience how success breeds success! Once a good relationship and rapport with a child or youth have been developed, a clear message should be sent, conveying confidence in their ability to take on large challenges. Given the above, the majority of time during a treatment session should be dedicated to *doing* exposures, not *discussing* exposures or the OCD ladder. If a therapist finds they are talking excessively about an exposure plan, it is possible that they or the child or youth is (either consciously or unconsciously) trying to stall and avoid. It is preferable to attempt an imperfect ERP and miss the mark a bit than to spend a session talking about (but not doing) an ERP.

Pitfall 5: Not Initially or Consistently Incorporating Meaningful Rewards

As discussed previously, it is important to have a well-thought-out and motivating reward system in place. Unfortunately, it is very common for this system to be underdeveloped and underestimated. It is preferable to start with a well-defined reward program at the beginning, with a plan to build in a discontinuation of rewards as sessions progress. Adding in a reward system in an attempt to make up for noncompliance or poor motivation part of the way through treatment is less effective than having the child or youth experience the positive reinforcement of rewards right from the beginning when the easiest ERPs are conducted. Parents may lose enthusiasm about providing rewards after their child has begun to make some progress on the OCD ladder, or they may promise to give the rewards at a later point in time. However, it is important that rewards be provided as promised as soon as possible following each attempted ERP. Delaying these until a later, undefined time point represents a lost opportunity to build the child or youth's confidence and motivation in their battle to boss back OCD.

Pitfall 6: Not Adjusting Homework after ERP Noncompliance

The converse of the expression "If it ain't broke—don't fix it" is "If it didn't work—try to fix it!" Children and youth do not always do what they are told, or what they say they will do! Often (very often) children and youth return to session not having completed their exposure homework. When that happens, the therapist *must* make changes to the homework for the next session. Never allow the child or youth to leave the office without making some kind of adjustment to the treatment plan. Even if they make proclamations such as "This week I'm really going to do it. I'll make time and you'll see. I'll practice every day," adjustments must be made. Why? Because something interfered with the child's homework completion, and that variable needs to be addressed. Possible variables include motivation, the difficulty of the ERP, the lack of support from parents to get it done, or insufficient time or opportunity.

There are two ways to make these modifications. The first approach involves lowering the bar on the valence of the ERP; in other words, modify the exposure such that less distress is evoked. The second approach involves keeping the exposure the same but introducing another adjustment. For example, an additional incentive could be negotiated or a plan can be made for a supportive person, like a parent or friend, to be present to coach the child or youth through this exposure, while holding the support person accountable for ERP completion. Chances are that if a child or youth did not complete a specific homework exposure on one occasion, then they will be unlikely to complete it the following week without some kind of change in the plan. Be sure to check in that the child or youth has access to the materials they need for specific exposures and that they have sufficient time to get them done.

Pitfall 7: Therapist Not Taking Responsibility for Unsuccessful ERPs

One of the most helpful therapeutic techniques when treating OCD is for the therapist to take the blame for the child or youth's difficulty in completing an exposure task. This technique helps to decrease the child's defensiveness and to prevent them from giving up altogether due to their lack of success. The following statement can help to keep a child or youth engaged for future ERPs:

> "I'm so sorry, I need to apologize. I gave you an ERP task that you weren't quite ready for yet. I misjudged and it's my fault that this didn't go quite as planned. Let's work together to think of a slightly different task that might be better for you right now."

Pitfall 8: Nonresponse Despite the Above

As with any treatment approach, clinicians will be faced with nonresponse in some instances, despite working through the previous modules and troubleshooting approaches, and having strong clinical skills! In these circumstances, taking a step back, reviewing the section above, and seeking informal or formal peer consultation may be of help. The worst thing to do is to keep doing the same thing and expecting something different to happen each time. Even the most seasoned OCD therapists will have clients who do not respond to planned ERPs. At these times, therapists may wish to consider adjunct therapists, such as ACT.

Pitfall 9: Distraction with Non-OCD Issues and Symptoms

Another pitfall is to get "distracted" by less impairing symptoms related to other disorders/behavior problems/small conflicts that happen between sessions. It is a good reminder not to lose the focus on treating OCD when other problems—as detailed on the next section—arise and do not require addressing in the moment.

Pitfall 10: Not Recognizing When to Stop

It is possible that previously unrecognized or newly emerging factors are interfering with success, which should be addressed before pushing forward with ERP. For example, if a recent family crisis such as a death in the family or home eviction occurs, this would be expected to markedly impact the ability of the youth and family to focus on OCD treatment.

As noted in the treatment preparation checklist, it is important to consider whether a comorbid condition or symptoms require stabilization or resolution before diving into ERP, given that stress levels and related maladaptive coping behaviors, such as cutting and other forms of self-injury will predictably worsen during treatment if not addressed prior to the start of ERPs. Similarly, some comorbid conditions, such as skin picking with resultant serious skin infections, and certain types of tics that could cause serious injury, may also worsen and detract from an ERP treatment plan.

It is also possible that the initially planned order of treatment for OCD and its comorbidities should be switched. As previously mentioned, medication management of depression prior to ERP initiation might improve conditions for success. However, if a diagnosis of depression emerges in the midst of ERP treatment, directly targeting this when it occurs may be necessary prior to continuing ERP.

Another common situation relates to ADHD comorbidity. In youth who are anxious, and particularly those who are susceptible to activation, a stimulant trial may result in markedly increased panic/agitation and subsequent discontinuation, while initial stabilization of OCD may lead to conditions under which stimulants are better tolerated. However, if ADHD-related hyperactivity and distractibility prevent CBT progress, then initial management of those symptoms may be preferable. Once the above factors have been addressed, consideration should be given to augmenting, complementary, or alternative treatment approaches for OCD (see Chapter 4).

Treatment-Interfering Behaviors

Sometimes, despite attempts to provide evidence-based therapy, children or youth fail to improve. There are certain behaviors that prevent full participation in treatment, thereby compromising its success. Alec Pollard at St. Louis Behavioral Medicine Institute refers to these as treatment-interfering behaviors (TIBs). According to Pollard, a TIB, is "any behavior that is incompatible or directly interferes with a person's ability to participate in therapy directly." For treatment to be successful it is important to assess the existence of TIBs and to address them.

The following are examples of such behaviors:

- Consistently failing to complete ERP homework
- Repeatedly missing sessions, either canceling or not showing up
- Engaging in behaviors that are not conducive to a session's progress, such as tantrums and aggression
- Using illicit substances
- Constantly debating and engaging the therapist in discussions about the validity of ERPs
- Presenting each week with a new peripheral crisis to address, derailing and distracting from the treatment focus
- Denying the existence of symptoms or downplaying their severity
- Refusing to talk or participate in the session

These behaviors need to be addressed in a systematic way before continuing with treatment. For more information about how to implement Pollard's approach, including a tool to aid in identifying TIBs, see Jonathan Grayson's (2014) book *Freedom from Obsessive–Compulsive Disorder: A Personalized Recovery Program for Living with Uncertainty* (2014).

Treatment Refusers

In training, clinicians are often advised that if an individual does not want to participate in therapy, then they cannot be forced. While this is true in certain respects, for families with a child or youth who is refusing treatment, throwing up one's hands and saying "there is nothing we can do" is not a viable option. The stakes are often high, and it is typically the entire family that is suffering due to the accommodations that have been made. When a child or youth refuses to participate in treatment, parents can still obtain help. Working with parents on limiting accommodations, dealing with challenging behaviors, and restoring some normalcy to daily life is critical. This is also important because when parents begin to pull back on OCD accommodations, the child or youth's motivation to engage in treatment may increase. For example, the child or youth might not think they have a problem because parents accommodate all of their OCD demands, such as buying excessive hygiene supplies and doing endless loads of laundry. It is not until those accommodations stop and the child or youth actually runs out of clothes that they may realize they need help in fighting OCD.

On a related note, when parents begin to pull back on accommodations, children or youth are initially very unhappy. This can result in emergence of challenging behaviors that parents need to deal with, including temper tantrums, screaming, and even physical aggression. Thus, it is critical for parents to have a therapist who can support them through this change. Finally, OCD often makes it challenging for parents to look after their own needs. Parents themselves have often compromised critical elements of self-care. They may be repeatedly late for work, chronically deprived of sleep as they are up all night to assist with rituals, eating poorly, and so forth. Parents often need reminders to put themselves

MODULE 7 HANDOUTS AND WORKSHEETS FOR PARENTS

Problem Solving Barriers to Success

The focus of today's treatment module is on taking risks. In other words, your child will begin to tackle the more distress-provoking ERPs at the top of their ladder. At this point in treatment, it is important that your child face the fears that were previously rated as 8 or higher on the OCD Ruler. Over the course of treatment, these ratings may have decreased but these exposures are still going to be viewed as very challenging by your child. We will introduce the concept of visualization to help children prepare themselves to do what only a few weeks ago was considered unimaginable.

The focus of today's parent materials is on problem solving difficulties you or your child may have encountered with ERPs.

Review of Material Covered in the Module 7 Handouts and Worksheets for Children and Youth

Visualization: Visualization has been used in sports for decades to prepare athletes for important games or matches. Visualization is the process of creating a mental image or intention of what you want to have happen or to feel. Mentally rehearsing the outcome of an event provides athletes with a heightened sense of well-being and confidence, which is associated with sports success. We can apply this same technique before attempting challenging ERP tasks. In session, children or youth are asked to identify a difficult ERP task on their ladder. Then they are asked to create a scenario in their mind in which they confront the obsessional trigger and successfully habituate to it. They will be asked to use all their senses: visual (images and pictures), kinesthetic (how the body feels), olfactory (what they smell), and auditory (what they hear). Once this exercise has been completed, your child should be ready to tackle their challenging ERP for real with the additional confidence that comes through visualization.

Barriers to Treatment Success

By Module 7, it is most likely that you will have seen your child make progress on at least some OCD symptoms. Like most families, you've also probably hit a few stumbling blocks with attempted ERPs. Some of the obstacles may have to do with the nature of the ERPs themselves (for example, too distressing, not disressing enough, practice is too infrequent); however, there are often challenges associated with the performance of the ERP that interfere with habituation and treatment success. Here is a list of problems, and possible solutions to keep your child moving forward with their ERPs:

Problem 1: Is your child replacing an old compulsion with a new one?

This is a very common problem. For example, your child may have reduced their handwashing but replaced it with avoidance or excessive checking of the cleanliness of their hands. The obsessional trigger has remained the same, as has the intrusive thought and the associated

(page 1 of 4)

From *OCD in Children and Adolescents: The "OCD Is Not the Boss of Me" Manual* by Katherine McKenney, Annie Simpson, and S. Evelyn Stewart. Copyright © 2020 The Guilford Press. Permission to photocopy this material is granted to purchasers of this book for personal use or use with children or youth and their parents (see copyright page for details). Purchasers can download additional copies of this material, in color (see the box at the end of the table of contents).

distress. The only thing that has changed is the nature of the ritual. OCD is sneaky and will try really hard to keep the distress and compulsions going. The solution is to be vigilant for signs of new compulsions and to incorporate these behaviors into ERPs. A related issue is the use of mental rituals during ERPs. This involves doing mental compulsions to prevent feared outcomes, which renders ERPs ineffective. Only your child knows if they are doing mental rituals, and your child's therapist should be regularly checking in during ERPs to see if this is something that needs to be addressed.

Problem 2: Is your child bailing out of ERPs too soon?

Some children terminate the ERPs before their anxiety level has decreased sufficiently. The general rule is that they should continue with the ERP until their anxiety has been reduced by half, although this is not always the case. If your child is ending an ERP too soon, they will be unable to habituate to the triggers. Even more concerning is the fact that ending an exposure task too soon and engaging in the ritual actually reinforces the symptom. It's as though the OCD is saying, "See, don't you feel so much better when you do what I tell you to?," which makes it more likely that the symptom will continue in the future.

Problem 3: Is your child's perfectionism interfering with ERPs?

Children and teens can be overly perfectionistic in their exposures, which can interfere with the successful completion of the ERP. For example, the child may be excessively monitoring their anxiety level to ensure they have achieved the "right" or "perfect" degree of anxiety. Similarly, the child may be trying so hard to create the perfect exposure that they have difficulties even getting started. If they feel the exposure is not being performed perfectly, it may be terminated prematurely. Emphasizing the importance of doing the exposure, rather than how well it is being performed, can be helpful.

Problem 4: Is your child blocking the experience of distress during ERPs?

The experience of distress is uncomfortable and unpleasant for youth to endure, so it is not uncommon for them to inadvertently or purposefully engage in behaviors or strategies to minimize the discomfort they experience during ERPs. There are several ways this can be accomplished:

- **Dulling:** Sometimes individuals try to shut out the experience of the exposure, thereby dulling themselves to the distress. This may involve dissociating themselves from the experience and telling themselves that "it's not me really doing this" as a way to handle their discomfort. This dulling/dissociation prevents the process of habituation from occurring. Therefore, it is important that children remain alert and connected to the distress throughout the exposure.
- **Distraction:** Children often use distraction techniques during ERPs to minimize the discomfort associated with them; this can include watching television, chatting with others, listening to music, etc. Not all distraction is bad and sometimes it is the only way children can initially resist engaging in compulsions/rituals. But for real habituation to occur, children must stay focused on the task at hand and fully experience the rise in their distress, as well as its inevitable decrease. Experiencing anxiety is the only way to truly get over anxiety. This means turning off the TV, pausing conversations, and turning off music during ERPs. It also means staying present in the situation where the ERP is occurring. Leaving the room after encountering an obsessional trigger and resisting a compulsion is much less effective than staying put and riding out the distress.

- **Safety signals:** Sometimes the mere presence of other people during ERPs can result in reduced anxiety. These safety signals can be obvious, such as when a parent repeatedly reminds the child that they are safe and that nothing bad will happen to them during ERPs. Sometimes these safety signals can be more covert. For example, if a child says, "I'm probably not going to get sick if I touch this, right?" Even parental silence can be interpreted as "Well, my mom didn't say anything so that must mean I'll be okay." In such subtle instances of reassurance-seeking, it may be more helpful to respond with "Maybe, maybe not. Let's see what happens."
- **Safety behaviors:** ERPs may fail to trigger sufficient anxiety if the child has already taken steps to prevent themselves from carrying out the feared act. For example, if a child has a fear of stabbing their mother, exposures at home may be less anxiety-provoking if all the knives and scissors have been stored away. Similarly, if a child is afraid of being poisoned by household cleaners, ERPs at home will be less stressful if all the toxic cleansers have been replaced with nontoxic environmentally friendly versions. These safety behaviors will prevent your child's anxiety from rising sufficiently high enough during imaginal exposures since safety precautions have already been taken.

Problem 5: Does your child not have sufficient time to complete exposures?

This is a complaint made by most children and teens in treatment: **I don't have time to do my exposures**. In some cases, these statements may reflect the child's own anxiety about performing ERPs or a lack of motivation. In other cases, children and teens simply do not have enough free time to set aside 60 minutes per day to work on the ERPs. The demands of school, sports, and other extracurricular activities often leave little time left in the day. Here are some suggestions to address this obstacle:

- Schedule time in advance over each week to work on ERPs so that there are clear expectations and arrangements made to accommodate these activities. Just as you set aside time for soccer practice, you set aside time for ERPs.
- Other families have had success with making daily screen time conditional on completion of ERP tasks.
- For those children and teens who participate in a number of activities each week, some find that they need to temporarily put these activities on hold to allow them sufficient time and energy to focus on treatment. That is a decision that each family must make on its own.

Secondary Gains Associated with OCD

Secondary gains are those external motivators that contribute to the maintenance of one's symptoms. In OCD, secondary gain usually occurs as a result of an accommodation that has been made by the family to help a child cope with OCD and prevent the child from experiencing distress. It is important to note that a child does not seek out secondary gain. Rather, it emerges spontaneously and unexpectedly during the course of the disorder. Examples of secondary gains may include things such as:

Decreased household responsibilities.

For example, the child no longer has to take out the garbage because of contamination fears. They get out of having to do an unpleasant task. Getting over this fear might mean having to resume this chore.

(page 3 of 4)

More parental attention or more time with parents.

Given the importance of parents in treatment success, parents often find themselves paying more attention to their child or spending more time with them as part of the treatment program. Younger children in particular find this extra parental attention very rewarding. Getting over OCD may mean that this extra attention ends.

Decreased academic expectations.

Given the impact OCD can have on schoolwork, many children require temporary accommodations, such as extra time on tests, reduced workload, etc. Similarly, parents may lower their expectations regarding their child's academic performance due to the struggles with OCD. Reducing one's symptoms may result in an end to the accommodations and a return to higher standards for school performance.

Because secondary gain is rewarding for your child, they may attempt to seek these gains at the expense of their well-being. There are several ways that parents can address the issue of secondary gain, such as the following:

1. Try to spend consistent time with your child outside of ERPs or other OCD-related behaviors.
2. To help your child realize that OCD does not entitle them to extra parental attention, try to spend an equal amount of time with your other children, if applicable.
3. If your child has specific interests or hobbies, develop an interest in these areas so that your child sees that special attention from parents can come through a variety of avenues, not just OCD.
4. If specific household responsibilities need to be temporarily reduced in order to manage anxiety, be sure to replace these chores with other less anxiety-provoking tasks. For example, if your child is unable to take out the trash, then this can be replaced with making beds. This strategy will also help to reduce sibling conflict that might emerge due to the inequality in household chores.

Is secondary gain something that might be impacting your child? If so, how might you address this over the next week?

MODULE 7 HANDOUTS AND WORKSHEETS FOR PARENTS

Parent Monitoring for Module 7

Each week, monitor the OCD behaviors you observe. These include specific rituals (for example, handwashing, checking), things your child avoids doing, and any OCD-related accommodations that your child requires. Estimate how often these behaviors occur per day and record your response to them (that is, your emotional and/or behavioral reaction). Please bring this sheet with you to the next session.

OCD behaviors (compulsions/avoidance/demands)	Estimated daily average	Parental response

From *OCD in Children and Adolescents: The "OCD Is Not the Boss of Me" Manual* by Katherine McKenney, Annie Simpson, and S. Evelyn Stewart. Copyright © 2020 The Guilford Press. Permission to photocopy this material is granted to purchasers of this book for personal use or use with children or youth and their parents (see copyright page for details). Purchasers can download additional copies of this material, in color (see the box at the end of the table of contents).

MODULE 7 HANDOUTS AND WORKSHEETS FOR PARENTS

Therapist Update for Module 7 (to bring to the next session)

Describe any new symptoms that you noticed over the past week:

_____
_____
_____
_____
_____

Describe any particularly challenging OCD situations that occurred over the week:

_____
_____
_____
_____
_____

Describe any successes that your child experienced over the week:

_____
_____
_____
_____
_____

Is there anything else that you think your child's therapist needs to know about the past week? If so, please describe:

_____
_____
_____
_____
_____

From OCD in Children and Adolescents: The "OCD Is Not the Boss of Me" Manual by Katherine McKenney, Annie Simpson, and S. Evelyn Stewart. Copyright © 2020 The Guilford Press. Permission to photocopy this material is granted to purchasers of this book for personal use or use with children or youth and their parents (see copyright page for details). Purchasers can download additional copies of this material, in color (see the box at the end of the table of contents).

MODULE 8

Self- and Family Care

Boosting Self-Esteem, Attending to Personal Needs, and Managing OCD in Schools

In order for a plant to grow, fundamental elements are necessary, including sunlight, water, and oxygen. Similarly, in order for therapy and exposures to be successful, certain elements must be present within the family. Therapists should attend to these elements during therapy to provide a context in which children and youth will succeed and flourish. This module addresses self-esteem and components of self-care including diet, exercise, and sleep that are important for all family members. It also addresses how to manage OCD to optimize chances for success in the school setting.

Self-care and identity development can be sidetracked in a child or youth who is responding to demands of OCD throughout crucial years of "growing up." They often quit well-loved sports and activities, avoid social situations, and forgo opportunities and challenges in the service of avoiding OCD triggers. Reminding a child or youth of their own strengths and characteristics outside of OCD is often crucial to prepare their "reentry" into an OCD-free life.

Moreover, parents who have been occupied by having their child's OCD needs diagnosed and addressed often neglect personal needs as individuals and as a couple. Polarization between parental responses to the child's OCD also adds to the challenges of maintaining family stability. As with most other areas of parenting, consistent communication and limit setting across time and between coparents is central to consolidating behavioral change regarding the child or youth's OCD.

Boosting the Child or Youth's Self-Esteem

OCD has a tendency to take over the lives of children and families. It demands attention, becomes all absorbing, dominates conversation, and overshadows positive life events. As a result, it can be hard to remember that the affected child is not solely defined by their OCD. OCD can make children and youth miss out on important activities that increase positive feelings about themselves, such as hanging out with friends, going to school, or participating in extracurricular activities. Moreover, even when they try to resist a compulsion and end up giving in, they often feel like a failure. All children and youth have strengths, qualities, and accomplishments that should be celebrated. Over time, the OCD can significantly and negatively impact evaluation of their own self-worth. Self-esteem often suffers. It is unsurprising that OCD and depression often coexist in the teen and adult years.

Activities in the rest of this module are aimed at helping children and youth to remember those things that are special about them which are independent of the OCD. Remind them that OCD is something they have, not something that they are. A slogan emerging in recent years on T-shirts and posters distributed by the International OCD Foundation drives home this point: "OCD is not an adjective."

Challenge the child or youth to think about and recognize the following areas:

1. Things that they like about themselves.
2. Things that people tend to compliment them about.
3. Things that make them feel proud of themselves.
4. Major accomplishments they have had and how they felt during these times.

Then have them remind themselves of these more positive views of themselves during moments when the OCD gets them down or has taken away their hope. These positive thoughts can help motivate children to continue with their ERPs and fight back against the OCD bully. As noted by many families who have lived through OCD-challenging years, the resiliency that the child or youth has developed in the process can become a major strength in future life challenges outside of OCD.

The creative self-esteem-boosting activities provided below can be selected based upon the developmental stage and interests of the child or youth. This list is in no way exhaustive and is meant to get the therapist's creative juices flowing!

- Create a self-esteem collage using cut-out magazine images symbolizing the child or youth's positive qualities, things they like about themselves and their accomplishments.
- Make an "All about Me" poster. Place a picture of the child or youth in the middle and have them decorate around it with positive qualities about themselves.
- Create a comic strip about a time when the child or youth was successful and felt proud.
- Play the "self-esteem game," which involves going back and forth between two individuals, saying positive statements about themselves as fast as they can. Collect a candy or small reward for each statement.
- Introduce the idea of a gratitude journal to the child or youth. Every night before going to bed they are asked to write three to five statements describing things they are grateful for that went well during the day.

- Create a memory concentration game with positive traits that you as the therapist have identified as representing the child or youth. Every time they make a match they have to tell a story that demonstrates that trait (e.g., athletic, intelligent).
- Have the child or youth come up with three examples of the following: things they are good at, things they like about their appearance, challenges they have overcome, accomplishments they are proud of, ways they have helped others, things that make them unique, and so forth.

Sample Dialogue

THERAPIST: Sanjay, today I want us to do something a little different. You have been working so hard on your exposures, so today I want to chat a bit about how you feel about yourself. OCD has this way of taking over kids' lives. It becomes all that the family talks about and deals with. It becomes hard to remember that you are not your OCD! Do you ever feel that way?

SANJAY: Yes, totally, sometimes I say I don't want to go somewhere, like the mall, and my parents say, "Sanjay, that is just your OCD talking." And I'm like, NO! It's not my OCD—I just don't like the mall.

THERAPIST: Yes, exactly! So let's talk a little about who you are . . . Sanjay . . . what kinds of things make you special? What do you like about yourself? What do people compliment you on? What are some things you have done that you are super proud of? Let's try to come up with three things for each of these.

SANJAY: Oh, I don't know, I can't really think of anything. Truth is, my OCD has sort of become my life. I can't even remember what I did before.

THERAPIST: Okay, I get that, Let's start with trying to remember the things you like. So you said before, you don't like the mall—so what activities do you enjoy?

SANJAY: Well, I really like soccer. I actually used to be on a team.

THERAPIST: Really? Soccer—so what position did you play?

SANJAY: I was striker—people actually used to say I was really good . . .

THERAPIST: Wonderful, so let's write that down—good at soccer . . . So, what kinds of qualities do you think a person needs to be good at soccer?

SANJAY: Well, they need to be coordinated, athletic, hardworking, a team player . . .

THERAPIST: Totally! Those are great qualities! Do any of these describe you? Let's write those down too.

Empowerment Activities

Fighting OCD is not easy. Often kids and youth need a little push to motivate them to initiate treatment and to continue on when the going gets tough. That's when empowerment activities can be very beneficial. Empowerment activities serve to build up their confidence to face the OCD bully despite associated challenges. The following presents some favorite empowerment activities for children and youth, although the possibilities are endless. Channeling personal interests when creating these activities really helps with buy-in.

Decisional Balance Sheet

This activity works very well for youth who need a little extra motivation to understand why they should work so hard. Have the youth divide a sheet into quarters. In each quarter have them write the (in this order): advantages of not working on the OCD, disadvantages of not working the OCD, disadvantages of working on the OCD, and advantages of working on the OCD. In this way, the youth can look at the arguments and be able to objectively see why working on OCD is the best option.

OCD Piñata

This activity is a fun way to build motivation with children and youth of all ages. Have them decorate a piñata with representations of their OCD triggers (e.g., scary words, pictures). Then have them demolish the piñata, representing how they plan to fight back against the OCD bully. Sometimes the destruction of the piñata may be used as a poignant part of an end of treatment during a graduation celebration.

How Life Will Be Better

Similar to the decisional balance sheet used with youth, younger children might benefit from making a list describing how OCD has messed things up for them in their lives (e.g., how it's kept them from having fun with their friends, doing well in school, and/or caused problems with their families). After this, they can be challenged to brainstorm how their life will look different once the OCD is gone (e.g., they will have more time to do fun things, less fighting at home).

Drawing a Picture or Making a Model of OCD out of Clay

Have the child or youth create an image of their OCD out of paper or with clay (this is separate from the activity in Module 1). Then as sessions and exposures progress, the child can pull or rip a piece off the picture or sculpture until there is no longer anything left. This provides a nice visual and concrete example of how the OCD is getting smaller and to reflect the growing benefits of fighting back.

OCD Funeral

Planning a funeral for the OCD can also be very empowering for children and youth. They can be asked to create a picture or object that represents the OCD. Then they can create an invitation to the funeral, write a eulogy, and bury the OCD representation to symbolize the death of the OCD that has been bullying them.

Writing a Letter to the OCD

In a similar manner to the other ideas listed above, have children and youth write a detailed letter to the OCD expressing their anger at how it has messed up their life and how they plan to get rid of it.

The above list should inspire therapists to empower and motivate children and youth to take back the control from OCD and to boss back the OCD bully!

Self-Care for Parents

Remind parents that they cannot look after their children or youth if they are not looking after themselves first. Have them think about the last commercial flight they took and remind them of the standard safety announcements prior to take off: "If you are traveling with a child or someone who requires assistance, secure your own oxygen mask first, and then assist the other person."

In other words, to effectively keep their child safe, parents need to *first* ensure their own well-being. If they pass out due to lack of oxygen, they clearly won't be in a position to help their child. The same principle applies in the treatment for OCD. Explain that this also has the benefit of modeling good self-care for their children, which is an important life skill for anyone, but especially for those trying to stay well and keep OCD at bay.

Parents often state that they know about the importance of self-care, but they have difficulties prioritizing themselves to make this happen. Try to have parents elaborate on obstacles interfering with taking time for themselves, and help them to problem-solve how these barriers can be removed or managed. Then help them to generate a plan for the next week when they will find daily time just for themselves (not their partner, children, or extended family). Explain that these actions do not have to be dramatic, lengthy, or expensive. In fact, regular small acts of self-care (e.g., 2 minutes of mindfulness, going for a walk, reading a magazine) can be very restorative. Have the parents write their goals in session, log their activities in the following week, and report back on their homework success. Similar to the need to adjust when a child has not completed ERP homework, it will be important to modify and persist in encouraging the parent to do their self-care homework for subsequent sessions.

In addition to the above, remind parents of the importance of central pillars of health including diet, exercise, and sleep. These are all necessary to maximize resilience and to help the parent and their child address OCD-related challenges.

Managing OCD in the School Setting

OCD not only impacts functioning in the home but also causes significant interference in the school setting as well. Families and school professionals should be aware of the following possible impacts of OCD:

- Difficulties with school attendance and chronic lateness due to time-consuming morning rituals.
- Fatigue and lack of sleep.
- Difficulty concentrating and following instructions due to the mental effort consumed by obsessions and rituals.
- Challenging behaviors such as noncompliance, arguments, or rage as children try to avoid triggers.
- Repeated reassurance seeking with teachers, for example, that the child understood the assignment or completed it correctly.
- Excessive requests for explanations about assignments.
- Repeated confessions of feared transgressions (e.g., cheating).
- Delays in work completion due to rereading and rewriting, excessive checking, or being triggered.
- Avoidance of certain things in the school setting such as bathrooms, touching books, specific people, or certain words.
- Assignments not being handed in or being late.
- Perfectionism and just-right feelings interfering with assignment completion.
- Frequent and/or lengthy bathroom visits due to handwashing.

The above list is in no way exhaustive, and it is important to remain on the lookout for how OCD symptoms may be impacting schooling. Children and youth spend a significant amount of their waking hours in the school setting, so effective treatment must address this setting as well. Encourage families to be open with the school about their child's condition. A formal system of communication between school and home can be helpful.

At times the development of an individualized education plan (IEP) may be warranted to define adaptations based upon the student's needs. Adaptations are teaching and assessment strategies especially designed to accommodate a student's needs in order to improve their learning outcomes in a subject or course and help them demonstrate their mastery of concepts. It is very important to recognize that adaptations within an IEP for OCD must be *temporary*. Gradual withdrawal of these is the goal in OCD, unlike in some other conditions such as ADHD and learning disabilities. The adaptations must be individualized for the specific child and their symptoms, since what might be helpful for one child (e.g., extended time on tests) may actually be harmful for another (e.g., may result in more checking behaviors). The following are examples of *temporary* accommodations that could be contained in an IEP for OCD:

- Extra time on assignments and tests.
- Reduced workload.
- Alternative response modes (e.g., typing, recording on an iPad) when writing is a challenge.
- Providing a time limit for homework.
- Grades for completed work while disregarding incomplete items.
- Quiet space for tests.
- Presentations done with an iPad, in a small group, or one-on-one with a teacher.

- External reminders such as alarms and checklists to keep children on track.
- A scribe.
- Seating according to needs.

Again, these accommodations should be reviewed regularly and withdrawn in a gradual fashion as OCD symptoms improve. Treatment homework should directly target exposures that contribute to the reduction of these accommodations. For example, if a child is asking many questions a day for clarification, they could be allowed a certain number of "question cards" that they can use each day. Any unused cards can be traded in for prizes. The number of cards is gradually reduced over time.

Homework Assignments

For Module 8, therapists can assign the following for youth and parents to complete at home before the next session:

For Youth

Practice at least 3 ERPs daily between sessions. These ERPs are developed in session and recorded on the ERP Home Practice for Module 8 worksheet.

For Parents

- Complete the Parental Tracking of Self-Care Activities worksheet.
- Complete the Parent Monitoring worksheet (parent observations of various compulsions, avoidance behaviors, and accommodations that the child requires, as well as estimated per-day average of each, and how parents responded).
- Complete the Therapist Update worksheet. This sheet allows parents to share with the child's therapist any new OCD symptoms that were observed over the week, any particularly challenging OCD situations the family encountered, any successes that the child experienced, and any other information parents feel would be helpful for the therapist to know. Therapists should ask parents to provide them with this completed sheet at the start of the next session so they can address specific issues as needed with the child or with the whole family together.

MODULE 8 HANDOUTS AND WORKSHEETS FOR CHILDREN OR YOUTH

Self-Esteem Booster

When you're fighting the battle against the OCD bully, it can seem like your whole life is about obsessions and compulsions. Sometimes it's all your family talks about. Some days you'll feel really successful in your fight to boss back the OCD bully, and some days it may feel that the bully is in control. On those harder days, it can be difficult to remember that you have other things going on in your life besides OCD.

It's important to know that you are more than the OCD. You have many positive qualities, and you've had major accomplishments in your life. To help you remember what's special about you that's outside of OCD, let's make a list:

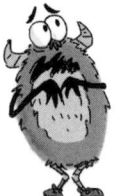 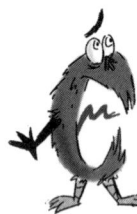 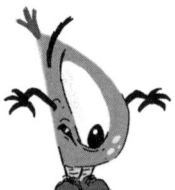

Things I like about myself: _____

_____

_____

_____

People tend to give me compliments about: _____

_____

_____

_____

_____

Things that make me feel proud of myself: _____

_____

_____

_____

_____

Remember, OCD is something you have, **not** who you are.

(page 1 of 3)

From *OCD in Children and Adolescents: The "OCD Is Not the Boss of Me" Manual* by Katherine McKenney, Annie Simpson, and S. Evelyn Stewart. Copyright © 2020 The Guilford Press. Permission to photocopy this material is granted to purchasers of this book for personal use or use with children or youth and their parents (see copyright page for details). Purchasers can download additional copies of this material, in color (see the box at the end of the table of contents).

The OCD Bully can make you feel really badly about yourself. Most kids feel bad about having OCD in the first place. If they try to resist a compulsion but end up giving in, then they can feel like a failure. Plus, the OCD bully can make people miss out on things that used to make them feel good about themselves, like hanging out with friends, doing well in school, or playing sports.

The important thing to remember is that it takes a lot of courage to get treatment for OCD. It's not an easy problem to get rid of, and you've come a long way in a short period of time. Remember, the OCD bully has been causing problems for you for months or even years and you've made progress in only a few weeks. Now, that's impressive.

What other things have you accomplished in your life (big or small)?

_____

_____

_____

_____

How did you feel when you succeeded in these things?

_____

_____

_____

_____

The next time you're faced with a difficult OCD situation or are struggling with a hard ERP, think back to all the success you've had in your life. Use this information to give you the confidence and strength to keep bossing back the OCD bully.

Now let's put that confidence to work while we spend the rest of the session practicing our ERPs . . .

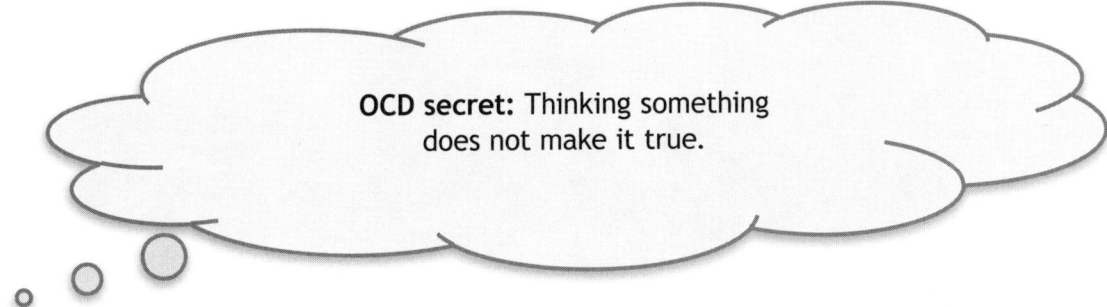

OCD secret: Thinking something does not make it true.

(page 2 of 3)

In-Session ERP Plan

ERP plan: _____

_____

_____

_____

_____

_____

OCD Ruler rating before the ERP: _____

OCD Ruler rating after the ERP: _____

Next steps? _____

_____

_____

_____

_____

_____

_____

_____

_____

_____

_____

_____

From *OCD in Children and Adolescents: The "OCD Is Not the Boss of Me" Manual* by Katherine McKenney, Annie Simpson, and S. Evelyn Stewart. Copyright © 2020 The Guilford Press. Permission to photocopy this material is granted to purchasers of this book for personal use or use with children or youth and their parents (see copyright page for details). Purchasers can download additional copies of this material, in color (see the box at the end of the table of contents).

MODULE 8 HANDOUTS AND WORKSHEETS FOR CHILDREN OR YOUTH

ERP Home Practice for Module 8

ERP task	Goal for the week	Daily homework results
		Day 1:
		Day 2:
		Day 3:
		Day 4:
		Day 5:
		Day 6:
	Reward:	Day 7:
		Day 1:
		Day 2:
		Day 3:
		Day 4:
		Day 5:
		Day 6:
	Reward:	Day 7:
		Day 1:
		Day 2:
		Day 3:
		Day 4:
		Day 5:
		Day 6:
	Reward:	Day 7:

From *OCD in Children and Adolescents: The "OCD Is Not the Boss of Me" Manual* by Katherine McKenney, Annie Simpson, and S. Evelyn Stewart. Copyright © 2020 The Guilford Press. Permission to photocopy this material is granted to purchasers of this book for personal use or use with children or youth and their parents (see copyright page for details). Purchasers can download additional copies of this material, in color (see the box at the end of the table of contents).

> MODULE 8 HANDOUTS AND WORKSHEETS FOR PARENTS

Self-Esteem, Self-Care, and Family Care

The focus of this treatment module is on fostering self-esteem. OCD often leaves young people feeling bad about themselves, partly because of the nature of the intrusive thoughts and ritualized behaviors, but also because OCD often results in children and youth missing out on things that previously made them feel good about themselves, such as school, sports, and spending time with friends. In this module, your child will be asked to think of positive qualities about themselves and reflect on past experiences when they have felt proud and accomplished.

The focus for parents in this module is on self-care. The treatment of OCD requires a tremendous amount of time and emotional resources from parents, often at the expense of their own well-being. This session will address the importance of self-care and how to dedicate time each week to foster parents' own needs.

Review of Material Covered in the Module 8 Handouts and Worksheets for Children or Youth

Self-esteem booster: The intrusive thoughts and compulsions found with OCD can have devastating effects that can undermine a child's self-esteem. This is particularly true for OCD-related perfectionism, as nothing ever feels "good enough." As well, those children who experience disturbing and taboo intrusive thoughts often think of themselves as horrible, disturbed people. Likewise, an inability to resist rituals or compulsions can lead people to consider themselves weak or a failure. The sensationalized media portrayals of individuals with OCD also do not contribute to your child's healthy sense of self. The internet is filled with memes, Buzfeed quizzes, and jokes about OCD that also result in OCD-affected youth feeling as though they, at best, are not understood, and at worst are an object of ridicule.

OCD and low self-esteem can form a vicious circle. Having OCD can make a child feel badly about themselves. In turn, low self-esteem makes it difficult for one to feel confident and capable of addressing OCD, which then further perpetuates the low sense of self-worth. Similarly, OCD often causes children and youth to withdraw from friends and other activities that previously contributed to positive self-esteem, such as achievements in academics or sports.

Fostering a positive sense of self is a gradual process. In session today, we begin that process by asking your child to identify the positive qualities and accomplishments of which they are proud. The message of the session is that OCD is something they have, not who they are. OCD does not have to define your child as a person. They have many qualities and skills that have nothing to do with OCD. This is frequently a difficult and uncomfortable task for young people, as they consider it bragging to identify their positive qualities. It is also very easy for us to think of things we don't like about ourselves; it's much harder to generate a list of things we do like about ourselves.

(page 1 of 2)

From *OCD in Children and Adolescents: The "OCD Is Not the Boss of Me" Manual* by Katherine McKenney, Annie Simpson, and S. Evelyn Stewart. Copyright © 2020 The Guilford Press. Permission to photocopy this material is granted to purchasers of this book for personal use or use with children or youth and their parents (see copyright page for details). Purchasers can download additional copies of this material, in color (see the box at the end of the table of contents).

Self-Care for Parents

OCD not only has an impact on how a family functions, but also on the well-being of individual family members. This is particularly true for parents. OCD can be quite draining on parents for a number of reasons:

- Children and teens may require ongoing parental reassurance.
- Parents are often directly involved in specific rituals.
- Rituals may interfere with parents' day-to-day functioning, making them late for work or distracted during other tasks.
- Bedtime and nighttime rituals can interfere with parents' own sleep (for example, parents may need to be present during night rituals; noise keeps parents awake).
- Parents experience heightened stress around how to parent a child with OCD.
- Parents experience increased worry and anxiety about their child's well-being.

In order to be an effective cheerleader in the child's battle against OCD, it is vital that parents be aware of the toll OCD can take on them, as well as of their own emotional needs. Parents often report that they feel selfish for taking time for themselves rather than focusing on their children. This sentiment is even more true in the case of OCD. In fact, the nature of OCD makes it even more important that parents maintain their full reserves of energy. The treatment of OCD requires a family approach, and you are going to need to draw on your energy resources in order to support your child effectively. You are more likely to remain patient and supportive when you are well rested and prioritizing time for yourself.

It is helpful to remember that a parent cannot look after their child if they are not looking after themselves first. Think about the last commercial flight you took. Do these safety instructions sound familiar?

If you are traveling with a child or someone who requires assistance, secure your own oxygen mask first, and then assist the other person.

In other words, to effectively keep your child safe, you need to **first** ensure your own safety. The same principle applies in the treatment for OCD. It is also helpful to know that it is good for your child to see you taking care of yourself because it gives your child permission to do the same.

The idea of taking care of oneself is not a novel concept, and many parents report already knowing the importance of self-care. If that's the case, then why is it so hard to put this idea into action? What gets in the way of taking time for yourself?

Over the next week, find time each day to do something just for you (not your partner or your children or your extended family). These actions do not have to be big, such as a weekend away. In fact, regular small acts of self-care can be just as restorative (for example, doing 2 minutes of mindfulness exercises, reading a book, going for a walk).

MODULE 8 HANDOUTS AND WORKSHEETS FOR PARENTS

Parental Tracking of Self-Care Activities

Day 1	Day 2	Day 3	Day 4	Day 5	Day 6	Day 7

From *OCD in Children and Adolescents: The "OCD Is Not the Boss of Me" Manual* by Katherine McKenney, Annie Simpson, and S. Evelyn Stewart. Copyright © 2020 The Guilford Press. Permission to photocopy this material is granted to purchasers of this book for personal use or use with children or youth and their parents (see copyright page for details). Purchasers can download additional copies of this material, in color (see the box at the end of the table of contents).

MODULE 8 HANDOUTS AND WORKSHEETS FOR PARENTS

Parent Monitoring for Module 8

Each week, monitor the OCD behaviors you observe. These include specific rituals (for example, handwashing, checking), things your child avoids doing, and any OCD-related accommodations that your child requires. Estimate how often these behaviors occur per day and record your response to them (that is, your emotional and/or behavioral reaction). Please bring this sheet with you to the next session.

OCD behaviors (compulsions/avoidance/demands)	Estimated daily average	Parental response

---

From *OCD in Children and Adolescents: The "OCD Is Not the Boss of Me" Manual* by Katherine McKenney, Annie Simpson, and S. Evelyn Stewart. Copyright © 2020 The Guilford Press. Permission to photocopy this material is granted to purchasers of this book for personal use or use with children or youth and their parents (see copyright page for details). Purchasers can download additional copies of this material, in color (see the box at the end of the table of contents).

MODULE 8 HANDOUTS AND WORKSHEETS FOR PARENTS

Therapist Update for Module 8
(to bring to the next session)

Describe any new symptoms that you noticed over the past week:

_____
_____
_____
_____
_____

Describe any particularly challenging OCD situations that occurred over the week:

_____
_____
_____
_____
_____

Describe any successes that your child experienced over the week:

_____
_____
_____
_____
_____

Is there anything else that you think your child's therapist needs to know about the past week? If so, please describe:

_____
_____
_____
_____
_____

From *OCD in Children and Adolescents: The "OCD Is Not the Boss of Me" Manual* by Katherine McKenney, Annie Simpson, and S. Evelyn Stewart. Copyright © 2020 The Guilford Press. Permission to photocopy this material is granted to purchasers of this book for personal use or use with children or youth and their parents (see copyright page for details). Purchasers can download additional copies of this material, in color (see the box at the end of the table of contents).

MODULE 9

Preparing for the Future
Relapse Prevention and Consolidating Gains

An important aspect of any treatment program is the incorporation of relapse prevention—taking steps to ensure the progress made in treatment is maintained after formal treatment ends. Help the child and their family to recognize the difference between a lapse and a relapse. A lapse is defined as a temporary return of symptoms, which may include a brief period of some intrusive thoughts and a return of compulsions or avoidance behaviors; however, the symptoms generally are not as impairing as the youth had experienced prior to treatment, and are usually easily ameliorated through an additional focus on ERPs. In contrast, a relapse is a worsening of symptoms consistent with pretreatment symptom severity. Prepare families for expected lapses in the future and discuss plans for addressing future symptom exacerbations so that lapses do not turn into relapses.

Early Warning Signs of Symptom Return

As OCD may sometimes follow a waxing and waning course across the life-span, it is important that families be aware of early signs of symptom exacerbations. The sooner they recognize that OCD has returned, the sooner they can implement previously learned strategies and possible booster sessions, thereby mitigating impairment and distress. This is not to suggest that parents, children, or youth should be overly vigilant of any potential sign of returning OCD. Rather, families should be mindful of the possibility of worsening OCD and to take note if they observe clusters of concerning behaviors. It's helpful for clinicians to inform families of the following potential early warning signs:

- Deteriorating academic performance
- Disordered sleeping (e.g., difficulties falling asleep, nighttime wakening)

- Avoidance of previously enjoyed activities
- Avoidance of specific people, situations, or objects
- Increased irritability and/or anxiety
- Requests for family members to change aspects of their daily routines
- Frequent/repetitive questions to family members
- New secrecy about specific activities

These are often specific early warning signs for different OCD symptom types. For example, a return of contamination fears could result in increasingly long showers, evidence of washing rituals (e.g., red/chapped hands, the need to frequently replenish cleaning products), or the subtle use of barriers. Clinicians can also help families to identify specific signs of symptom exacerbations that are unique to the child or youth's symptom presentation.

When to Anticipate Potential Symptom Exacerbations

It can be empowering for children, youth, and families to understand that, despite the fact that symptoms may return, these exacerbations can often be anticipated, which allows for early intervention. Times to anticipate some recurrence of symptoms include any periods of stress. This could include a negative stressor (e.g., a death, or family breakup) but also more neutral or positive experiences of stress (e.g., transitions such as holidays or graduation). Fatigue, illness, and transitions to new developmental stages can also be points of vulnerability. Entry into adolescence with its associated hormonal and life shifts is also a period when OCD flares can occur. At these times, an increase or new onset of intrusive thoughts can be expected.

It is important for families to recognize that a return of symptoms should not evoke panic, as this does not necessarily indicate full relapse. Remind the family that they will be in a very different position compared to the initial onset of OCD, as they will have the tools to fight it and prevent it from taking over their lives.

Consolidating Gains

One of the most important aspects of relapse prevention is the consolidation of gains that were made over the course of treatment. In terms of the "OCD Is Not the Boss of Me" treatment program, this refers to the ability of the child or youth and parent to apply skills learned in developing ERPs for a variety of symptom presentations. Doing so will allow family members to demonstrate their understanding of ERPs and their ability to construct effective exposures, and, most importantly, it will help them to prepare for future OCD exacerbations that may differ from current OCD symptoms. Below are a number of activities to help consolidate the learning that has taken place during treatment.

- Provide fictional scenarios of a child or youth with OCD whose symptoms are different from those addressed in treatment. Have them describe a variety of ERPs that

this fictional child or youth could complete, as well as how to structure them in a gradual way.
- A variation on this technique is for the clinician to write "Dear Abby" letters asking for advice in the voice of a child or youth who has OCD. Then have them respond to the letter, conveying hope, empathy for the child or youth's experience, and suggestions for ERPs that could be helpful.
- Have the child or youth write a letter that you will give to the next individual you will help with OCD (being respectful of confidentiality, of course). Have them describe how they felt at the start of treatment, what was learned, including ERPs, how life has changed, and their hopes for your next child or youth.
- For those who are willing, record them speaking to future OCD-affected children and youth about their own experience in treatment and the benefits of ERP.

Sample Dialogue

THERAPIST: So, Luca, I'm so proud of all you have accomplished over the last 3 months. You really kicked OCD to the curb! I'm so impressed with how you were able to take the tools and boss back your OCD! It would be super helpful if you could write a letter about your journey to the next kid who I am going to see, describing what you learned and giving any advice you might have for them. What do you say? You wouldn't put your name on it, so they wouldn't know who you are if you don't want.

LUCA: Sure, that sounds good.

Sample Letter

Dear kid with OCD,

I know how you feel—it's pretty scary when you start OCD treatment. When I started I couldn't even leave my room. I had stopped going to school—hadn't been there in a month! I washed my hands all the time and they were all cracked and bleeding. I even had Lysol wipes to wipe down everything in my room if anyone came in! I look back now and think to myself—wow, how did I let OCD boss me around so much? I want to tell you that you can boss it back—it doesn't have to rule your life. It was so hard at first, but the candy and prizes did make it easier. The 4 S's really help—I especially liked sillying it and shrinking it. Exposures are really the most important thing to help you get better. So my advice to you is to do the exposures! Stay focused on the rewards at first (I really liked money, to be honest). But with time, it just feels so good to get your life back—to be the boss again. Nobody likes a bully—and OCD is such a bully! You can do this!!!

Preparing for Graduation

As the second to last module, preparations for the end of treatment should be incorporated into this session. We will often ask children or youth how they would like to mark their last session in terms of special treats or activities to celebrate their progress to date. We also ask them to complete a special homework project that encourages them to creatively reflect on their symptoms' improvements, or what it has been like to suffer from OCD, or how life feels different now. There are no specific rules so encourage them to focus on a medium (for example, video, painting, photographs, a collage, a poster, a poem, a short story) that is meaningful for them. Parents are typically present when children or youth show their project in the next session, so it's helpful for them to know that in advance in case that impacts what they choose to do.

Photographs of some projects that children have completed over the years to help inspire therapists and youth appear on below and on pages 215–216.

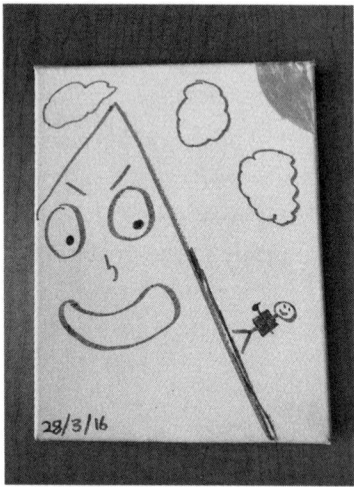

PHOTO 1. A painting by a 10-year-old showing the youth climbing up the OCD mountain, illustrating that he's on his way toward conquering his OCD.

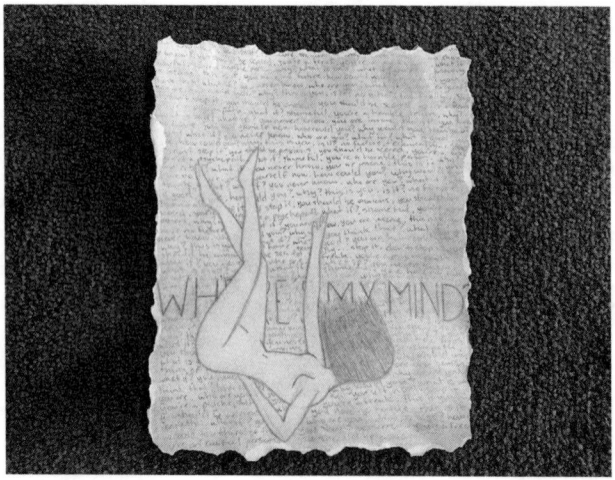

PHOTO 2. A drawing by a 14-year-old that illustrates how lost and overwhelmed she felt by her intrusive thoughts before treatment.

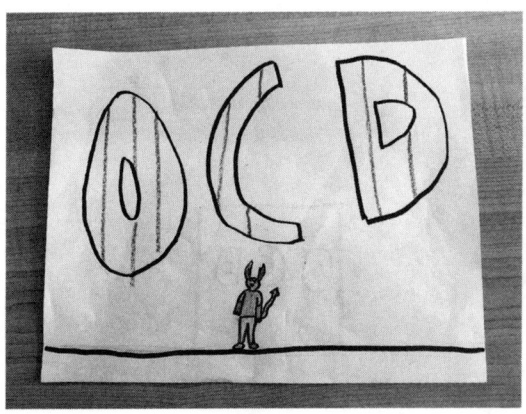 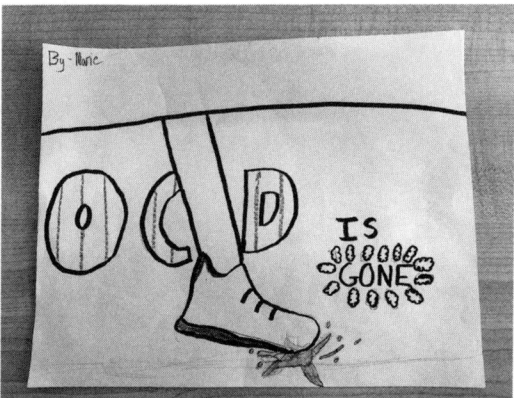

PHOTO 3. An 11-year-old's drawing of her OCD before treatment (left), and after treatment (right).

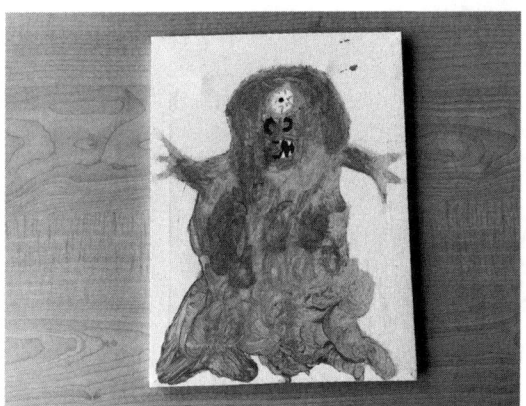 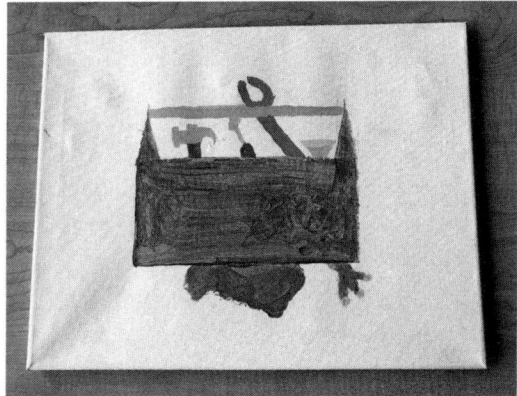

PHOTO 4. A 15-year-old's painting of his OCD before treatment (left; note that his eyes, nose, and mouth spell "OCD"), and his OCD after treatment (right; squished by all the strategies in his toolbox).

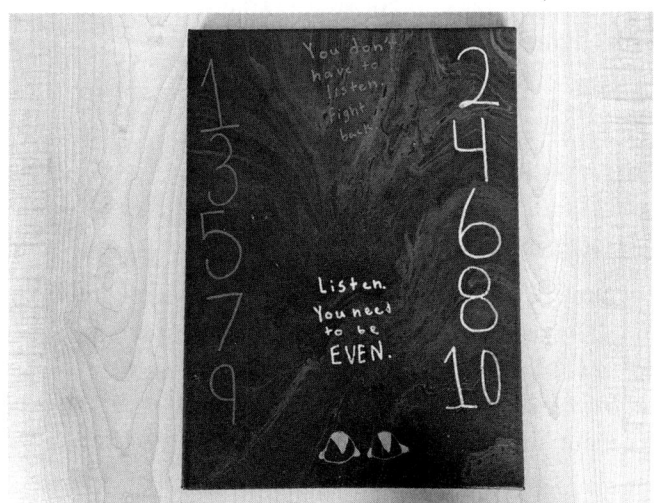

PHOTO 5. A painting by a 9-year-old that illustrates OCD's need for things to be even, and how she bosses the OCD back.

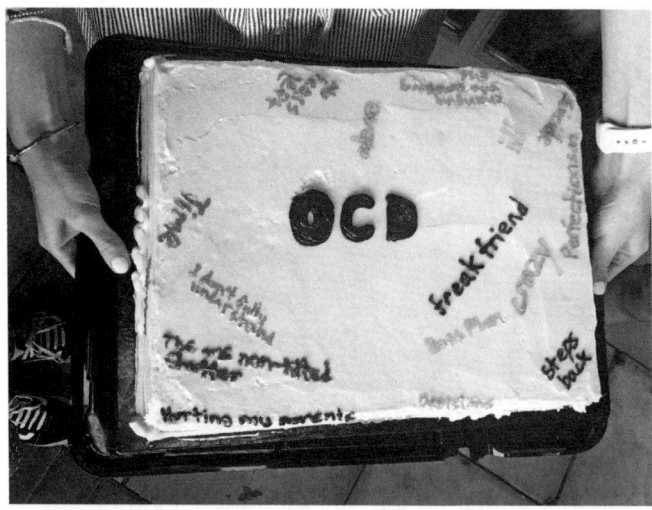

PHOTO 6. A cake decorated by a 15-year-old that shows various OCD-trigger words, descriptions of how OCD made him feel, and rituals he used to complete. At graduation, he then smashed the cake (which was enjoyed by family and the therapist).

Homework Assignments

For Module 9, therapists can assign the following for youth and parents to complete at home before the next session:

For Youth

- Practice at least 3 ERPs daily between sessions. These ERPs are developed in session and recorded on the ERP Home Practice for Module 9 worksheet.
- Create a project that reflects the child or youth's treatment journey, how life has changed, or what life was like living with OCD.

For Parents

- Complete the Parent Monitoring worksheet (parent observations of various compulsions, avoidance behaviors, and accommodations that the child requires, as well as estimated per-day average of each, and how parents responded).
- Complete the Therapist Update worksheet. This worksheet allows parents to share with the child's therapist any new OCD symptoms that were observed over the week, any particularly challenging OCD situations the family encountered, any successes that the child experienced, and any other information parents feel would be helpful for the therapist to know. Therapists should ask parents to provide them with this completed worksheet at the start of the next session so they can address specific issues as needed with the child or with the whole family together.

MODULE 9 HANDOUTS AND WORKSHEETS FOR CHILDREN OR YOUTH

Preparing for the Future

After completing eight modules, you've hopefully experienced some major changes in your life and with your OCD. At this point, some kids aren't bothered by the OCD bully anymore while others still have some obsessions and compulsions that they are working on. Either way, you've made major progress, and you should be really proud of what you've accomplished so far.

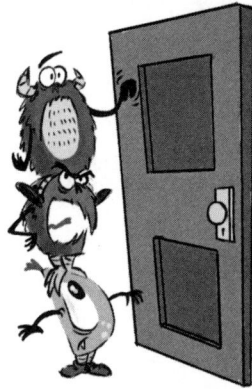

There's one pesky detail about the OCD bully that is important to remember: the OCD bully tends to come and go and you need to be prepared to boss back the bully in the future, even if he's gone now. That's just the way it is. You can go through long periods of time without being bothered by an OCD thought or by feeling the need to do a ritual, but then, out of the blue, the OCD bully can come knocking on your door. It may be a new obsession or it might be something you've dealt with in the past. Either way, the return of OCD symptoms can be really frustrating and alarming to kids. They might think, *"Oh no, it's back again. It's going to be just like before."*

The good news is that you're a very different person now then you were when the OCD bully first showed up and took over your life. Think about how you're different and write it down.

_____

_____

_____

_____

_____

_____

Hopefully you remembered that you've learned tricks to manage your OCD. Now you know that OCD is nothing more than a bully that you can send packing by using the strategies in your backpack.

(page 1 of 4)

From *OCD in Children and Adolescents: The "OCD Is Not the Boss of Me" Manual* by Katherine McKenney, Annie Simpson, and S. Evelyn Stewart. Copyright © 2020 The Guilford Press. Permission to photocopy this material is granted to purchasers of this book for personal use or use with children or youth and their parents (see copyright page for details). Purchasers can download additional copies of this material, in color (see the box at the end of the table of contents).

When the OCD bully makes its next uninvited appearance into your life, it's important to remember the following things:

- OCD is not going to be as bad as before because now you know what it is and what to do about it.
- It doesn't mean that you've failed.
- It doesn't mean that all your hard work in this program was for nothing. OCD comes and goes. That's just the way the illness works.
- Just because the bully is back, it doesn't mean it's back forever.

In fact, a full relapse is very unlikely because you've got a team of people supporting you in your fight against the OCD bully; and you've also got a backpack full of strategies. The good news is that the bully won't stick around for long because this program has taught your brain to react differently to OCD thoughts and its tricks.

So if the OCD bully starts causing problems again, here are some things to **do** and **not do**:

1. **Do** tell your parents that you think OCD is trying to sneak its way back in. They can help you to boss it back.
2. **Do** talk to your therapist. You may just need a booster session.
3. **Do** review the strategies in your binder. You may just need a refresher.
4. **Don't** pretend it isn't happening.
5. **Don't** ignore it and hope that the OCD bully will go away.
6. **Don't** keep it a secret.

Since we know it's highly likely the OCD bully will try to come back at some point, let's see if we can beat OCD at its own game. Let's try gazing into our crystal ball and imagine where the OCD bully might show its ugly head in the future. Write down a situation and the obsession/compulsion that you might be faced with in the future.

_____

_____

_____

_____

_____

_____

_____

_____

(page 2 of 4)

What strategies in your backpack could you use to show the OCD who's boss in the future?

_____
_____
_____
_____
_____
_____
_____

What ERP could you do to deal with this obsession/compulsion?

_____
_____
_____
_____
_____
_____
_____

Part of overcoming OCD is acknowledging that it comes and goes and being ready for when the OCD bully shows up on your doorstep. And when it does . . . slam the door in its face! How do you do that? By recognizing an OCD thought for what it is (a bully in your brain), remaining calm, and using a strategy to get rid of it. Remember, it's nothing to panic about. It's just a sign that you need to do something about it.

Time for more practice . . .

(page 3 of 4)

In-Session ERP Plan

ERP plan: _____

_____

_____

_____

_____

_____

OCD Ruler rating before the ERP: _____

OCD Ruler rating after the ERP: _____

Next steps? _____

_____

_____

_____

_____

_____

_____

_____

_____

_____

_____

MODULE 9 HANDOUTS AND WORKSHEETS FOR CHILDREN OR YOUTH

It's Time to Get Creative

You've been on an incredible journey. When you started this program, the OCD bully was running your life and causing all kinds of problems for you and your family. Now you know how to boss back the OCD bully and get control over your life. That's an amazing change!

When you go through major life changes, it's important to take a moment and reflect back on the process and how life is different for you. Sometimes the best way to do this is by being creative.

For homework this week, you're going to create something that expresses your experience of coping with OCD. It's up to you how you want to do this. Here are some ideas to help you get started:

- Poem
- Drawing or painting
- Short story
- Song or rap
- Video
- Collage
- Cartoon
- Poster
- Model or clay figurine
- Papier-maché artwork
- Photographs
- Diorama

There is no right or wrong way to do this assignment. Do something that will be fun and meaningful for you. Bring your project with you to the next session to show your therapist and parents. Most importantly, have fun doing this!

From *OCD in Children and Adolescents: The "OCD Is Not the Boss of Me" Manual* by Katherine McKenney, Annie Simpson, and S. Evelyn Stewart. Copyright © 2020 The Guilford Press. Permission to photocopy this material is granted to purchasers of this book for personal use or use with children or youth and their parents (see copyright page for details). Purchasers can download additional copies of this material, in color (see the box at the end of the table of contents).

MODULE 9 HANDOUTS AND WORKSHEETS FOR CHILDREN OR YOUTH

ERP Home Practice for Module 9

ERP task	Goal for the week	Daily homework results
		Day 1:
		Day 2:
		Day 3:
		Day 4:
		Day 5:
		Day 6:
	Reward:	Day 7:
		Day 1:
		Day 2:
		Day 3:
		Day 4:
		Day 5:
		Day 6:
	Reward:	Day 7:
		Day 1:
		Day 2:
		Day 3:
		Day 4:
		Day 5:
		Day 6:
	Reward:	Day 7:

From *OCD in Children and Adolescents: The "OCD Is Not the Boss of Me" Manual* by Katherine McKenney, Annie Simpson, and S. Evelyn Stewart. Copyright © 2020 The Guilford Press. Permission to photocopy this material is granted to purchasers of this book for personal use or use with children or youth and their parents (see copyright page for details). Purchasers can download additional copies of this material, in color (see the box at the end of the table of contents).

MODULE 9 HANDOUTS AND WORKSHEETS FOR PARENTS

Relapse Prevention and Future Planning

The focus of today's treatment session is on relapse prevention. Relapse prevention involves techniques that are designed to anticipate triggers for a reemergence of OCD symptoms in the future. For many children and youth, a return of OCD symptoms at some point in their lives is highly likely. The good news is that they have learned strategies they can use to boss back any new symptoms fairly quickly.

The focus for parents in this module is on preparing for the future, both in terms of celebrating successes to date and learning how to address OCD once treatment has ended.

Review of Material Covered in the Module 9 Handouts and Worksheets for Children or Youth

The following concepts are presented:

Relapse prevention: Most children do not want to consider the possibility of a relapse (that is, when OCD makes a significant and persistent return despite a child's best efforts at symptom management). It is more helpful to think of the return of OCD as a "brain blip," a brief and unexpected symptom exacerbation which unfortunately, is a fairly common part of the course of OCD. This not only helps children prepare themselves for the possibility of future OCD symptoms, but also helps them react to them more adaptively. These future brain blips are not an indication of failure, nor do they mean that all the gains made in treatment have been lost. Rather, future brain blips are part of the disorder. The good news is that these are usually time-limited and can be dealt with. By using the strategies taught in this program, children can prevent these brain blips from turning into relapses. One relapse prevention technique is to reinforce the internalization of the CBT techniques learned in the program. To do this, your child will be asked to imagine a future brain blip and how they would design an ERP to face the fear, as well as identify other techniques they could use (for example, Bossing Back OCD").

The importance of informing others about symptoms: If and when a future brain blip emerges, the most important thing children and teens can do is to tell someone about it, whether it's their parents or therapist. It is not helpful to ignore the symptoms and to hope they will go away on their own. Most children have already tried that tactic with minimal success. In fact, ignoring the symptoms enables the OCD to become more consolidated and, therefore, more challenging to address. The sooner a child discloses information about future brain blips, the sooner a strategy can be implemented to deal with the OCD symptoms.

Preparing for graduation: The next module will be the final one, and a portion of that will be spent on celebrating your child's accomplishments since they began the program. Your child will take time in session to plan their graduation (for example, special treats, activities). As part of their graduation, both the therapist and parents will be invited to speak about the changes they have witnessed in the child over the course of the program. Please take a moment before

(page 1 of 2)

From *OCD in Children and Adolescents: The "OCD Is Not the Boss of Me" Manual* by Katherine McKenney, Annie Simpson, and S. Evelyn Stewart. Copyright © 2020 The Guilford Press. Permission to photocopy this material is granted to purchasers of this book for personal use or use with children or youth and their parents (see copyright page for details). Purchasers can download additional copies of this material, in color (see the box at the end of the table of contents).

the next session to think about what you want to say about your child. These comments should focus on the gains and progress that have been made, rather than on obstacles and barriers encountered over the course of treatment or on what remains to be done.

Parents' Role in Relapse Prevention

Parents play a key role in relapse prevention by remaining alert and vigilant for the emergence of new (or reemergence of old) OCD symptoms, particularly during times of stress. So what should parents do if they suspect OCD may be returning after treatment has ended?

1. Don't panic! Remember, these brain blips are a natural part of the disorder and should not come as a surprise.
2. Determine if your child is aware that OCD may be returning.
3. Don't protect your child from stress and triggers in order to minimize the symptoms.
4. Collaboratively begin ERP activities to address these symptoms. Reviewing these materials is also helpful. Consider contacting your child's therapist for a booster session.

Children who have completed treatment often complain that their parents become "OCD police" and constantly attribute their behaviors and actions to OCD. While you as a parent need to be alert for the potential of future OCD symptoms, there is a fine line between being vigilant and becoming intrusive by constantly asking, "Is that OCD?" One way to manage this balancing act is to establish a weekly OCD check-in with your child. As the name implies, this involves sitting down once a week and checking in on the frequency and severity of symptoms, as well as inquiring about behaviors you have observed over the week that you suspect may be OCD. These meetings allow for an open discussion about symptoms and enable a child to receive necessary supports.

Medication and Progess

If children are also taking medication to treat the OCD, it is important that they recognize that **they** are responsible for the gains made in treatment. It is their hard work that has resulted in a reduction of OCD symptoms. Medication merely allows a child to more fully engage in the treatment process by turning down the volume of the symptoms.

MODULE 9 HANDOUTS AND WORKSHEETS FOR PARENTS

Parent Monitoring for Module 9

Each week, monitor the OCD behaviors you observe. These include specific rituals (for example, handwashing, checking), things your child avoids doing, and any OCD-related accommodations that your child requires. Estimate how often these behaviors occur per day and record your response to them (that is, your emotional and/or behavioral reaction). Please bring this sheet with you to the next session.

OCD behaviors (compulsions/avoidance/demands)	Estimated daily average	Parental response

From *OCD in Children and Adolescents: The "OCD Is Not the Boss of Me" Manual* by Katherine McKenney, Annie Simpson, and S. Evelyn Stewart. Copyright © 2020 The Guilford Press. Permission to photocopy this material is granted to purchasers of this book for personal use or use with children or youth and their parents (see copyright page for details). Purchasers can download additional copies of this material, in color (see the box at the end of the table of contents).

MODULE 9 HANDOUTS AND WORKSHEETS FOR PARENTS

Therapist Update for Module 9 (to bring to the next session)

Describe any new symptoms that you noticed over the past week:

_____
_____
_____
_____
_____

Describe any particularly challenging OCD situations that occurred over the week:

_____
_____
_____
_____
_____

Describe any successes that your child experienced over the week:

_____
_____
_____
_____
_____

Is there anything else that you think your child's therapist needs to know about the past week? If so, please describe:

_____
_____
_____
_____
_____

From OCD in Children and Adolescents: The "OCD Is Not the Boss of Me" Manual by Katherine McKenney, Annie Simpson, and S. Evelyn Stewart. Copyright © 2020 The Guilford Press. Permission to photocopy this material is granted to purchasers of this book for personal use or use with children or youth and their parents (see copyright page for details). Purchasers can download additional copies of this material, in color (see the box at the end of the table of contents).

MODULE 10

Graduation

Celebration and Maintenance of Gains

Reflecting on Progress and Identifying Residual Symptoms

As treatment nears its end, it is important to take time to reflect on the progress that has been made. It is often helpful to have children or youth review the symptoms they identified in the worksheets from Module 1 so they can see how far they have come. Many times, they will remark that they are surprised at what they can do now or that they never thought they would get over a specific symptom. And while not everyone experiences a significant decline in all of their symptoms, most can at least identify broader changes such as decreased stress in the family household, a better understanding of OCD among family members, and an increased ability to tackle OCD in the future.

Although active treatment may be drawing to a close, that does not mean that children, youth, and families should stop conducting ERPs. ERP practice is a key part of the next phase of treatment: maintenance of treatment gains. Clinicians should alert children, youth, and families to the need for ongoing ERPs, although, depending on the number and intensity of residual symptoms, the frequency of needed ERP practice will vary.

To identify symptoms that families should continue to target once active treatment is over, clinicians should help children, youth, and their parents complete the table in Module 10 on page 231. Completing this table allows children and youth to identify the OCD symptoms that were present at the start of treatment and then reflect on whether the symptoms have worsened, improved, or resolved over the course of treatment. They can also identify whether any particular symptoms have remained unchanged. Those compulsions and obsessions that have either worsened or have not yet responded to treatment should be the focus of ongoing ERPs.

Follow-Up Booster Sessions and Maintenance

After a successful course of treatment, many children, youth, and families feel ambivalent about coming to the end of therapy. While they may be excited about the additional free time and a decrease in daily ERP practice, they may also have anxiety about coping with OCD symptoms without weekly or regular clinical sessions. This anxiety can be alleviated in several different ways. Once a child or youth is exhibiting steady progress in treatment and the clinician is confident in the family's understanding of the treatment model, sessions can be gradually spaced out so that a family starts attending biweekly, and then eventually monthly, sessions.

Families (and most often children and youth) ask at the end of treatment, "Do I have to keep doing my ERPs?" And the answer is "Yes," although the frequency of the ERPs can change during the maintenance phase of treatment. When working with a therapist weekly in active treatment, families should aim to complete 30–60 minutes of homework ERPs per day. Once in the maintenance phase of treatment, families can decrease the amount of time spent in ERPs on a daily basis, as the purpose is to maintain gains already made in treatment. There is no magic number, but families should aim to complete at least one ERP per day. And the frequency of these per day will decrease further as the child continues to make progress and is no longer bothered by specific obsessions or engaging in certain rituals.

It can also be helpful for families to be offered booster sessions as required. The opportunity to meet with a clinician again for a review of treatment strategies and to develop new ERPs can be invaluable. In our experience, one or two booster sessions during a period of symptom exacerbation is typically sufficient to reengage the family in the practice of ERPs and to boost their confidence in their ability to manage symptoms independently.

Graduation: Celebratory Activities

The treatment journey is almost complete! The final session is an opportunity to acknowledge progress and celebrate success. Although the final session is an opportunity to recognize symptom improvement, youth often like to mark their success with other celebratory activities outside of session with their families. Have youth identify how they would like to celebrate—some youth choose going out for dinner, others request a party complete with cake, while others opt to celebrate by accomplishing a task that they previously avoided or were unable to do (e.g., see a movie in the theatre in seats that are never cleaned.) Have youth also identify a meaningful person (outside of their parents) with whom they can share their treatment progress with. This kind of disclosure not only helps to address residual stigma and secrecy, but serves as another opportunity for children and youth to receive positive feedback and praise for all their hard work.

Take time in your session with children/youth and parents together for the child to present their special homework assignment from last session. This project, regardless of what the child or youth elects to do, should express their experience of coping with OCD and how life has changed for them. We find that these are some of the most powerful moments in treatment, as it allows another outlet for youth to reflect on their progress and to express their feelings about treatment in a way that is meaningful for them. Occasionally, youth do not complete this assignment for the final session. In those situations, we will often ask the child or youth to talk a bit about what life was like when OCD was at its worst, what can they do now they couldn't do before, what was most helpful in treatment, and so on. Therapists may have to ask some leading questions to guide the child and youth through this portion of the session. This is also an opportunity for the parents and the therapist to share their experience of supporting the child and the child's strengths. We typically suggest that the therapist speak after the parents to "repair" any comments that may detract from the celebration of progress (e.g., "Imagine how much better you could be if you'd just tried harder in therapy.")

Although formal and regular treatment sessions may be ending, youth and parents should leave with the understanding that ongoing ERP practice will most likely still be required. Emphasize that they have the skills necessary to address OCD symptoms and encourage them to "lean into" the OCD rather than avoid triggers when they arise. Encourage the family to celebrate the successes to date. As part of termination, you can provide your client with a graduation certificate (see p. 233).

MODULE 10 HANDOUTS AND WORKSHEETS FOR CHILDREN OR YOUTH

You've Come a Long Way!

Whew! It's been a lot of hard work, but you did it! You have completed the program, learned how to boss back the OCD bully, and taken back control over your life. Congratulations! You should be really proud of yourself. Big achievements like this should be celebrated.

How do you want to celebrate your accomplishment?

_____
_____
_____
_____

It's important to share your good news. Identify someone who knows about your struggle with OCD who you can share this accomplishment with.

_____

You learned a lot since you started. What strategies were the most helpful for you?

_____
_____
_____
_____

What was life like before this program? How is life different for you now?

_____
_____
_____
_____
_____

(page 1 of 3)

From *OCD in Children and Adolescents: The "OCD Is Not the Boss of Me" Manual* by Katherine McKenney, Annie Simpson, and S. Evelyn Stewart. Copyright © 2020 The Guilford Press. Permission to photocopy this material is granted to purchasers of this book for personal use or use with children or youth and their parents (see copyright page for details). Purchasers can download additional copies of this material, in color (see the box at the end of the table of contents).

Do you remember on the very first day of this program when you wrote down the obsessions and compulsions that were causing you problems? Let's look back over this list and see what's changed since then. Write down the obsessions and compulsions and make a check mark to show whether they have gotten worse, stayed the same, improved, or even disappeared since the program started.

Obsessions	Gotten worse	No change	Improved	Disappeared

Compulsions	Gotten worse	No change	Improved	Disappeared

Based on this information, what obsessions and/or compulsions still need some work?

_____

_____

_____

How will you work on these in the coming months?

_____

_____

_____

(page 2 of 3)

Just for fun . . . let's do some more ERPs.

Exposure task	Goal	Results

A final thought . . .

                        You've done it.

          Keep using the strategies in your backpack.

                          Remember,

OCD IS NOT THE BOSS OF YOU!

CONGRATULATIONS

_____
(name)

has successfully completed the
"OCD is Not the Boss of Me"
program

on

_____
(date)

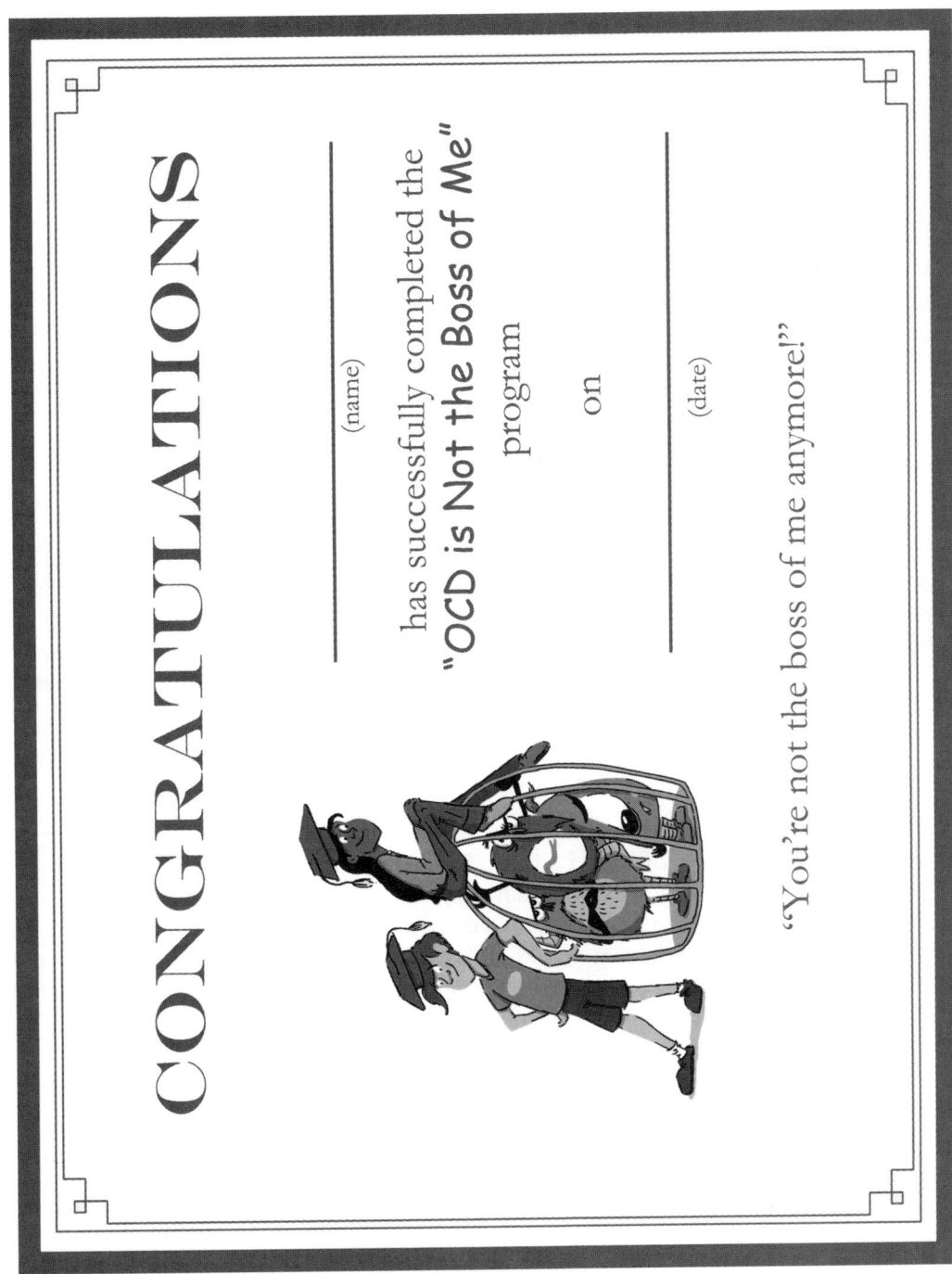

"You're not the boss of me anymore!"

From *OCD in Children and Adolescents: The "OCD Is Not the Boss of Me" Manual* by Katherine McKenney, Annie Simpson, and S. Evelyn Stewart. Copyright © 2020 The Guilford Press. Permission to photocopy this material is granted to purchasers of this book for personal use or use with children or youth and their parents (see copyright page for details). Purchasers can download additional copies of this material, in color (see the box at the end of the table of contents).

MODULE 10 HANDOUTS AND WORKSHEETS FOR PARENTS

Graduation

The focus of this module is on celebrating . . . celebrating your child's progress, celebrating their new confidence in managing OCD, and celebrating the end of OCD bossing them around. This is also a time to celebrate the work parents have done in learning to tolerate their child's OCD-related distress and to decrease accommodation. At the end of this standardized treatment program, some children's symptoms will be in remission, while others will still require "bossing back" on a daily basis. Regardless of the severity and frequency of your child's symptoms, they are now in a position to continue to fight back against their OCD and reclaim their lives.

For parents the focus of this module is also on preparing for the future, both in terms of celebrating successes to date and in addressing long-term management of OCD once this phase of therapy has ended. This includes discussion of topics such as future treatment, preparing to discontinue medication if applicable, and ongoing ERPs.

Review of Material Covered in the Module 10 Handouts and Worksheets for Children or Youth

The following concepts are presented:

Celebrating accomplishments: In this module your child's progress will be celebrated with treats, a graduation ceremony, and a certificate. The certificate serves as a tangible reminder of the strategies and skills your child has learned. Your child will also be asked to think about how else they would like to mark the occasion of completing the program. Common examples are dinner at a restaurant, a family outing, or a reward of some kind. As long as these things are within reason (and within budget), it is important to do what you can to ensure that these requests are honored.

Informing others about progress: Your child will be asked in session to identify a person who is at least somewhat aware of their OCD and with whom they can share their treatment gains. Notifying trusted others is a concrete way of solidifying progress made in therapy. In other words, "saying it out loud makes it real." While some children will be reluctant to share their experiences with others, they are encouraged to identify at least one person who can celebrate their progress. From a child's perspective, it never hurts to get praise and positive reinforcement from a close friend or extended family member. It also further eliminates the secrecy that OCD thrives on.

Symptom review: Your child will be asked to recall their first session and to think about how their identified symptoms have changed (that is, worsened, unchanged, improved, disappeared). This review helps to put into perspective how far your child has come in such a short period of time (and how worthwhile it has been to give up the time required for OCD treatment!).

(page 1 of 3)

From *OCD in Children and Adolescents: The "OCD Is Not the Boss of Me" Manual* by Katherine McKenney, Annie Simpson, and S. Evelyn Stewart. Copyright © 2020 The Guilford Press. Permission to photocopy this material is granted to purchasers of this book for personal use or use with children or youth and their parents (see copyright page for details). Purchasers can download additional copies of this material, in color (see the box at the end of the table of contents).

Acknowledging your own accomplishments as a parent

Although the focus of this module is primarily on the progress your child has made, it is important to acknowledge how far you as a parent have come in terms of your understanding of OCD and how to best support your child. Your new attitude and approach to OCD have been critical in your child's success. Moreover, your commitment to regularly come to sessions has sent several important messages to your child:

- that their well-being is of the utmost importance to you
- that getting over OCD is a priority
- that they are not alone in the battle against OCD

Take a moment to congratulate yourself and pat yourself on the back for a job well done! Even if your child has remaining OCD symptoms, they will be encouraged to continue bossing back their OCD, knowing that you as their parent are right beside them.

Looking ahead to the future

Your family now has an opportunity to practice managing your child's OCD without regular therapist check-ins. You and your child know everything you need to know in order to manage OCD effectively. We encourage you to regularly review the materials from both the child and parent modules and to set weekly targets for ERPs. You will find blank copies of many of the worksheets as well as a summary of the strategies taught, and the OCD secrets, to help you and your child review what you have learned.

Ongoing ERP . . . the work never stops

Just because the treatment program has ended, it does not mean that the work has ended. In fact, now the real work begins! You and your child will need to continue to work on ERP tasks on a daily basis in order to keep OCD at bay. Your child may not require the intensity of ERP tasks that were assigned during the active program; however, daily practice of at least one ERP per day will not only ensure that your child maintains the gains from treatment, but will also better prepare them for the inevitable future brain blips.

So what is the secret for making sure OCD becomes nothing more than background noise for the rest of your child's life? Children need to make sure they keep bossing back the OCD. The key is to make this response second nature so that they are automatically able to identify any future brain blips and disregard these as OCD thoughts that do not make sense, that are not grounded in reality, and that are not important (rather than becoming upset after interpreting the brain blips as something significant or predictive).

What to expect

It is very common for children to experience a rebound of OCD symptoms after treatment ends. This is usually attributed to the absence of regular sessions that concentrate on symptoms, as well as an absence of therapist-assigned ERP tasks. OCD symptom rebound at treatment termination is expected and a well-documented phenomenon, and is not something that should cause inordinate parental concern.

Things to consider if your child plans to stop taking medication

If your child is taking medication for their OCD and has experienced significant improvement, you may be wondering about discontinuing the medication. This is a decision that should be made in consultation with your prescribing physician.

Here are a few things to consider:

- Every child is unique and determining how long to remain on medication is a personal decision that depends on a number of factors. Research with adults suggests that taking these medications for about a year has been associated with a lower rate of relapse.
- When the time comes to gradually taper off the medication, booster sessions with a therapist can be helpful.

A Final Note

Thank you for all of your hard work and for refusing to allow OCD to take over your family's life anymore. It's been a difficult journey, and may be one that is still in progress. But together with the strategies you've learned and your resolve to no longer give in to OCD's demands, you have what you need to keep OCD from robbing your child of their future plans and goals. Job well done!

Strategies in My Backpack

Here are all the strategies you learned in this program:

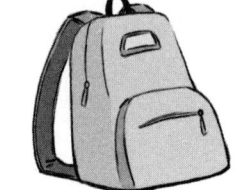

1. OCD Ruler
2. Catch the OCD bully
3. Exposure and response prevention
4. Escaping the OCD bully's trap
5. Bossing back the OCD bully
6. Imaginal exposures
7. Worry script
8. Making an appointment with OCD
9. Shift it
10. Shrink it
11. Switch it up
12. Silly it
13. Floating on by
14. Coping cards
15. Coping with Doubt script

Are there other strategies that you've thought of on your own? Write them down:

_____
_____
_____
_____
_____
_____
_____

From *OCD in Children and Adolescents: The "OCD Is Not the Boss of Me" Manual* by Katherine McKenney, Annie Simpson, and S. Evelyn Stewart. Copyright © 2020 The Guilford Press. Permission to photocopy this material is granted to purchasers of this book for personal use or use with children or youth and their parents (see copyright page for details). Purchasers can download additional copies of this material, in color (see the box at the end of the table of contents).

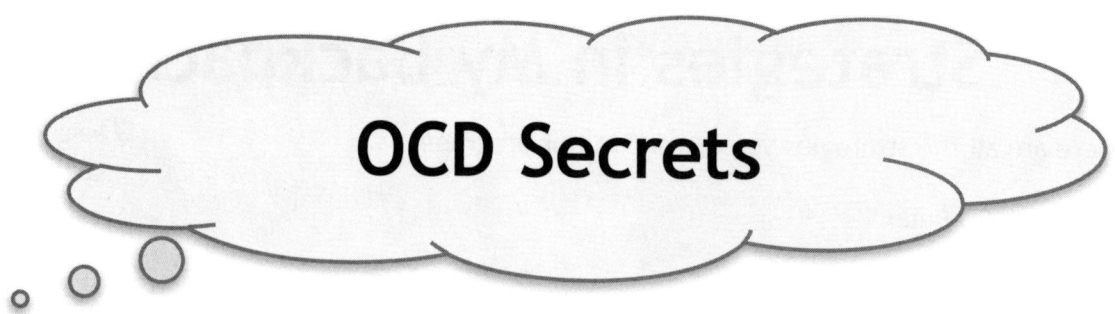

OCD Secrets

Here are all the OCD secrets you learned in this program:

1. Every time you stand up to the OCD bully, it gets a little smaller.

2. To get rid of OCD, you need to do the opposite of what OCD is telling you.

3. Our bodies are built to cope with anxiety.

4. OCD is a liar. You can't trust what it says.

5. Thoughts are just ideas. They are not reality.

6. Thinking something does not make it true.

Are there other OCD secrets that you've thought of? Write them down:

_____
_____
_____
_____
_____
_____
_____
_____
_____
_____

From *OCD in Children and Adolescents: The "OCD Is Not the Boss of Me" Manual* by Katherine McKenney, Annie Simpson, and S. Evelyn Stewart. Copyright © 2020 The Guilford Press. Permission to photocopy this material is granted to purchasers of this book for personal use or use with children or youth and their parents (see copyright page for details). Purchasers can download additional copies of this material, in color (see the box at the end of the table of contents).

OCD Ladder

OCD RULER

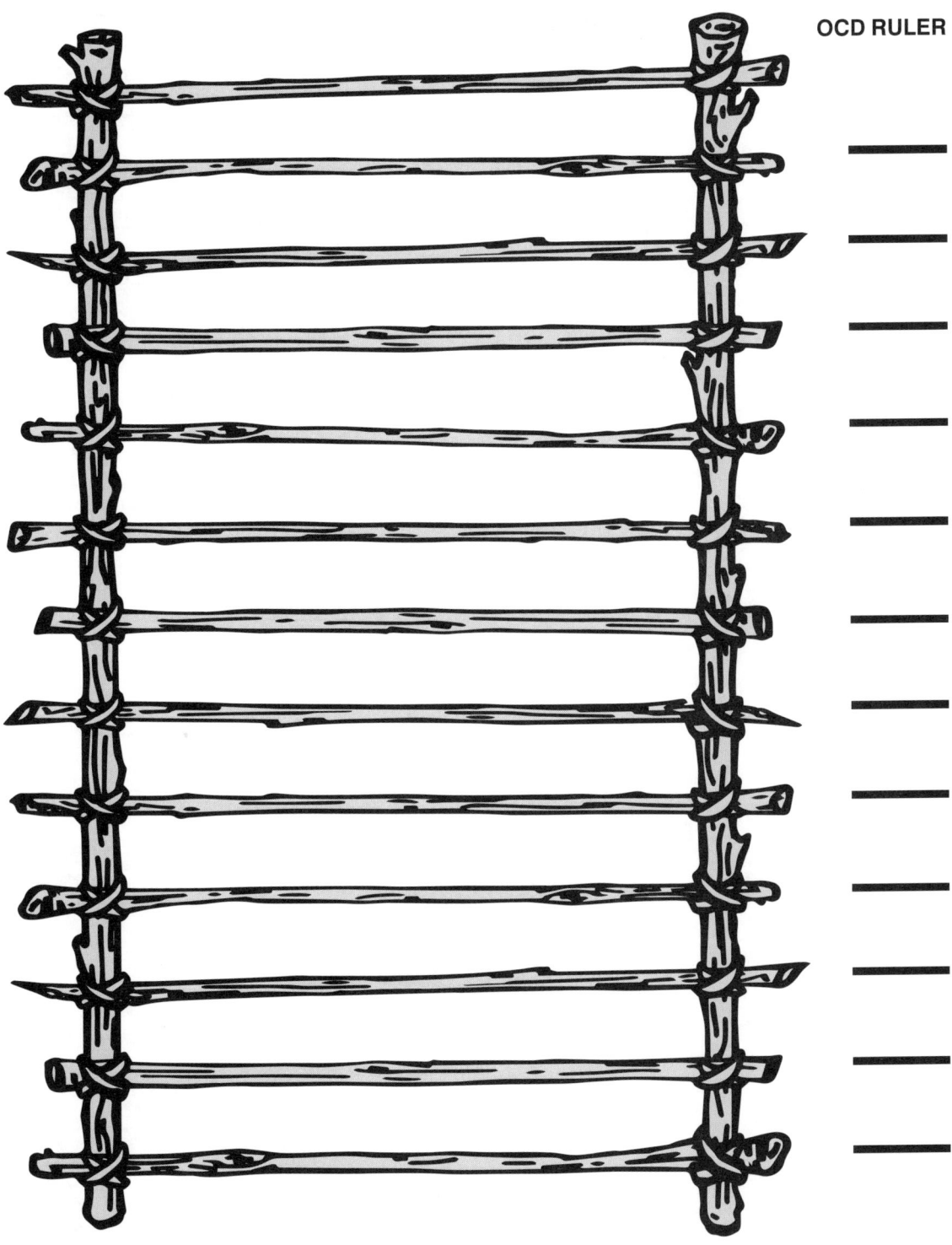

From *OCD in Children and Adolescents: The "OCD Is Not the Boss of Me" Manual* by Katherine McKenney, Annie Simpson, and S. Evelyn Stewart. Copyright © 2020 The Guilford Press. Permission to photocopy this material is granted to purchasers of this book for personal use or use with children or youth and their parents (see copyright page for details). Purchasers can download additional copies of this material, in color (see the box at the end of the table of contents).

ERP Home Practice

ERP task	Goal for the week	Daily homework results
		Day 1:
		Day 2:
		Day 3:
		Day 4:
		Day 5:
		Day 6:
	Reward:	Day 7:
		Day 1:
		Day 2:
		Day 3:
		Day 4:
		Day 5:
		Day 6:
	Reward:	Day 7:
		Day 1:
		Day 2:
		Day 3:
		Day 4:
		Day 5:
		Day 6:
	Reward:	Day 7:

From *OCD in Children and Adolescents: The "OCD Is Not the Boss of Me" Manual* by Katherine McKenney, Annie Simpson, and S. Evelyn Stewart. Copyright © 2020 The Guilford Press. Permission to photocopy this material is granted to purchasers of this book for personal use or use with children or youth and their parents (see copyright page for details). Purchasers can download additional copies of this material, in color (see the box at the end of the table of contents).

Escaping the OCD Bully's Trap Practice

Situation: _____

Feelings:
_____

Obsession

_____
_____
_____
_____
_____

(OCD Bully's Trap)

Compulsion/Avoidance

_____
_____
_____
_____
_____

Now try breaking free from the OCD bully's trap!

Feelings:
_____

Realistic Thoughts

_____
_____
_____
_____
_____

(Escaping the OCD Bully's Trap)

Realistic Behavior

_____
_____
_____
_____
_____

From *OCD in Children and Adolescents: The "OCD Is Not the Boss of Me" Manual* by Katherine McKenney, Annie Simpson, and S. Evelyn Stewart. Copyright © 2020 The Guilford Press. Permission to photocopy this material is granted to purchasers of this book for personal use or use with children or youth and their parents (see copyright page for details). Purchasers can download additional copies of this material, in color (see the box at the end of the table of contents).

References

Alvarenga, P. G., Cesar, R. C., Leckman, J. F., Moriyama, T. S., Torres, A. R., Bloch, M. H., et al. (2015). Obsessive–compulsive symptom dimensions in a population-based, cross-sectional sample of school-aged children. *Journal of Psychiatric Research, 62*, 108–114.

Bloch, M. H., Craiglow, B. G., Landeros-Weisenberger, A., Dombrowski, P. A., Panza, K. E., Peterson, B. S., et al. (2009). Predictors of early adult outcomes in pediatric-onset obsessive–compulsive disorder. *Pediatrics, 124*(4), 1085–1093.

Bloch, M. H., Landeros-Weisenberger, A., Kelmendi, B., Coric, V., Bracken, M. B., & Leckman, J. F. (2006). A systematic review: antipsychotic augmentation with treatment refractory obsessive–compulsive disorder. *Molecular Psychiatry, 11*(7), 622–632.

Bloch, M. H., Landeros-Weisenberger, A., Rosario, M. C., Pittenger, C., & Leckman, J. F. (2008). Meta-analysis of the symptom structure of obsessive–compulsive disorder. *American Journal of Psychiatry, 165*(12), 1532–1542.

Bloch, M. H., & Storch, E. A. (2015). Assessment and management of treatment-refractory obsessive–compulsive disorder in children. *Journal of the American Academy of Child and Adolescent Psychiatry, 54*(4), 251–262.

Bridge, J. A., Iyengar, S., Salary, C. B., Barbe, R. P., Birmaher, B., Pincus, H. A., et al. (2007). Clinical response and risk for reported suicidal ideation and suicide attempts in pediatric antidepressant treatment: A meta-analysis of randomized controlled trials. *JAMA, 297*(15), 1683–1696.

Chabane, N., Delorme, R., Millet, B., Mouren, M., Leboyer, M., & Pauls, D. (2005). Early-onset obsessive–compulsive disorder: A subgroup with a specific clinical and familial pattern? *Journal of Child Psychology and Psychiatry, 46*(8), 881–887.

Coelho, J. S., Zaitsoff, S. L., Pullmer, R., Franco Yamin, D., Anderson, S., Fernandes, A., et al. (2019). *Eating disorder and obsessive–compulsive symptoms—body checking in eating and obsessive–compulsive disorders: Exploration of shared vulnerability in a pediatric sample*. Manuscript submitted for publication.

Coluccia, A., Ferretti, F., Fagiolini, A., & Pozza, A. (2017). Quality of life in children and adolescents with obsessive–compulsive disorder: A systematic review and meta-analysis. *Neuropsychiatric Disease and Treatment, 13*, 597–608.

Craske, M. G., Treanor, M., Conway, C. C., Zbozinek, T., & Vervliet, B. (2014). Maximizing exposure therapy: An inhibitory learning approach. *Behaviour Research and Therapy, 58*, 10–23.

Cromer, L., Kaier, E., Davis, J., Stunk, K., & Stewart, S. E. (2017). Obsessive–compulsive disorder in college athletes. *American Journal of Psychiatry, 174*(6), 595–597.

De Wit, S. J., Van Der Werf, Y. D., Mataix-Cols, D., Trujillo, J. P., Van Oppen, P., Veltman, D. J., et al. (2015). Emotion regulation before and after transcranial magnetic stimulation in obsessive compulsive disorder. *Psychological Medicine, 45*(14), 3059–3073.

Dougherty, D. D., Brennan, B. P., Stewart, S. E., Wilhelm, S., Widege, A. S., & Rauch S. L. (2018). Neuroscientifically informed formulation and treatment planning for patients with obsessive–compulsive disorder: A review. *JAMA Psychiatry, 75*(10), 1081–1087.

Fayad, S. M., Guzick, A. G., Reid, A. M., Mason, D. M., Bertone, A., Foote, K. D., et al. (2016). Six–nine year follow-up of deep brain stimulation for obsessive–compulsive disorder. *PLOS ONE, 11*(12), e0167875.

Fineberg, N. A., Dell'Osso, B., Albert, U., Maina, G., Geller, D., Carmi, L., et al. (2019). Early intervention for obsessive compulsive disorder: An expert consensus statement. *European Neuropsychopharmacology, 29*(4), 549–565.

Flament, M. F., Whitaker, A., Rapoport, J. L., Davies, M., Berg, C. Z., Kalikow, K., et al. (1988). Obsessive compulsive disorder in adolescence: An epidemiological study. *Journal of the American Academy of Child and Adolescent Psychiatry, 27*(6), 764–771.

Flessner, C. A., Sapyta, J., Garcia, A., Freeman, J. B., Franklin, M. E., Foa, E., et al. (2011). Examining the psychometric properties of the Family Accommodation Scale-Parent–Report (FAS-PR). *Journal of Psychopathology and Behavioral Assessment, 31*, 38–46.

Foa, E. B., & Kozak, M. J. (1986). Emotional processing of fear: Exposure to corrective information. *Psychological Bulletin, 99*, 20–35.

Geller, D., Biederman, J., Faraone, S. V., Frazier, J., Coffey, B. J., Kim, G., et al. (2000). Clinical correlates of obsessive compulsive disorder in children and adolescents referred to specialized and non-specialized clinical settings. *Depression and Anxiety, 11*(4), 163–168.

Geller, D. A., Biederman, J., Stewart, S. E., Mullin, B., Martin, A., Spencer, T., et al. (2003). Which SSRI?: A meta-analysis of pharmacotherapy trials in pediatric obsessive–compulsive disorder. *American Journal of Psychiatry, 160*(11), 1919–1928.

Geller, D. A., & March, J. (2012). Practice parameter for the assessment and treatment of children and adolescents with obsessive compulsive disorder. *Journal of the American Academy of Child and Adolescent Psychiatry, 51*(1), 98–113.

Grayson, J. (2014). *Freedom from obsessive–compulsive behavior: A personalized recovery program for living with uncertainty* (updated ed.). New York: Penguin.

Guy, W. (1976). *Assessment manual for psychopharmacology, revised* (DHEW Publication ABM 76-366). Washington, DC: U.S. Government Printing Office.

Guy, W. (1997). *Clinical global impressions.* Rockville, MD: National Institute of Mental Health.

Hezel, D. M., & Simpson, H. B. (2019). Exposure and response prevention for obsessive–compulsive disorder: A review and new directions. *Indian Journal of Psychiatry, 61*(Suppl. 1), S85–S92.

Hezel, D. M., Stewart, S. E., Riemann, B., & McNally, R. (2019). Standard of proof and intolerance of uncertainty in obsessive–compulsive disorder and social anxiety disorder. *Journal of Behavior Therapy and Experimental Psychiatry, 64*, 36–44.

Hollander, E., & Wong, C. M. (1995). Obsessive–compulsive spectrum disorders. *Journal of Clinical Psychiatry, 56*(Suppl. 4), 3–6.

Ivarsson, T., Skarphedinsson, G., Kornør, H., Axelsdottir, B., Biedilæ, S., Heyman, I., et al. (2015). The place of and evidence for serotonin reuptake inhibitors (SRIs) for obsessive compulsive disorder (OCD) in children and adolescents: Views based on a systematic review and meta-analysis. *Psychiatry Research, 227*(1), 93–103.

Jaspers-Fayer, F., Han, S. H. J., Chan, E., McKenney, K., Simpson, A., Boyle, A., et al. (2017). Prevalence of acute-onset subtypes in pediatric obsessive–compulsive disorder. *Journal of Child and Adolescent Psychopharmacology, 27*(4), 332–341.

Jaspers-Fayer, F., Lin, S. Y., Belschner, L., Mah, J., Chan, E., Bleakley, C., et al. (2018). A case-control study of sleep disturbances in pediatric obsessive–compulsive disorder. *Journal of Anxiety Disorders, 55*, 1–7.

Kendall, P. C., Robin, J., Hedtke, K., Suveg, C., Flannery-Schroeder, E., & Gosch, E. (2005).

Considering CBT with anxious youth?: Think exposures. *Cognitive and Behavioral Practice, 12*, 136–150.

Lebowitz, E. R., & Omer, H. (2013). *Treating childhood and adolescent anxiety: A guide for caregivers.* Hoboken, NJ: Wiley.

Lebowitz, E. R., Omer, H., Hermes, H., & Scahill, L. (2014). Parent training for childhood anxiety disorders: The SPACE Program. *Cognitive and Behavioral Practice, 21*(4), 456–469.

Lebowitz, E. R., Omer, H., & Leckman, J. F. (2011). Coercive and disruptive behaviors in pediatric obsessive–compulsive disorder. *Depression and Anxiety, 28*, 899–905.

Lewin, A. B., Peris, T. S., Lindsey Bergman, R., McCracken, J. T., & Piacentini, J. (2011). The role of treatment expectancy in youth receiving exposure-based CBT for obsessive–compulsive disorder. *Behaviour Research and Therapy, 49*(9), 536–543.

McKenney, K. S. (2012). *Camp oh-see-dee: An intensive cognitive-behavioral therapy program for kids and teens with OCD.* Unpublished manual, Vancouver, Canada.

Melin, K., Skarphedinsson, G., Skärsäter, I., Haugland, B. S. M., & Ivarsson, T. (2018). A solid majority remit following evidence-based OCD treatments: A 3-year naturalistic outcome study in pediatric OCD. *European Child and Adolescent Psychiatry, 27*(10), 1373–1381.

Micali, N., Heyman, I., Perez, M., Hilton, K., Nakatani, E., Turner, C., et al. (2010). Long-term outcomes of obsessive–compulsive disorder: Follow-up of 142 children and adolescents. *British Journal of Psychiatry, 197*(2), 128–134.

Murphy, T. K., Gerardi, D. M., & Leckman, J. F. (2014). Pediatric acute-onset neuropsychiatric syndrome. *Psychiatric Clinics of North America, 37*, 353–374.

Naesström, M., Blomstedt, P., & Bodlund, O. (2016). A systematic review of psychiatric indications for deep brain stimulation, with focus on major depressive and obsessive–compulsive disorder. *Nordic Journal of Psychiatry, 70*(7), 483–491.

Negreiros, J., Belschner, L., Selles, R., Lin, S. Y., & Stewart, S. E. (2018). Academic skills in pediatric obsessive–compulsive disorder. *Annals of Clinical Psychiatry, 30*(3), 185–195.

O'Kearney, R. T. (2007). Benefits of cognitive behavioural therapy for children and youth with obsessive compulsive disorder: Re-examination of the evidence. *Australian and New Zealand Journal of Psychiatry, 41*(3), 199–212.

O'Kearney, R., Gibson, M., Christensen, H., & Griffiths, K. M. (2006). Effects of a cognitive behavioural internet program on depression, vulnerability to depression and stigma in adolescent males: A school-based controlled trial. *Cognitive Behaviour Therapy, 35*(1), 43–54.

Patel, S. R., Galfavy, H., Kimeldorf, M. B., Dixon, L. B., & Simpson, H. B. (2017). Patient preferences and acceptability of evidence-based and novel treatments for obsessive–compulsive disorder. *Psychiatric Services, 68*(3), 250–257.

Pediatric OCD Treatment Study Team. (2004). Cognitive-behavior therapy, sertraline, and their combination for children and adolescents with obsessive–compulsive disorder: The Pediatric OCD Treatment Study (POTS) randomized controlled trial. *JAMA, 292*(16), 1969–1976.

Pérez-Vigil, A., Fernández de la Cruz, L., Brander, G., Isomura, K., Jangmo, A., Feldman, I., et al. (2018). Association of obsessive–compulsive disorder with objective indicators of educational attainment: A nationwide register-based sibling control study. *JAMA Psychiatry, 75*(1), 47–55.

Peris, T. S., Bergman, R. L., Langley, A., Chang, S., McCracken, J. T., & Piacentini, J. (2008). Correlates of accommodation of pediatric obsessive–compulsive disorder: Parent, child, and family characteristics. *Journal of the American Academy of Child and Adolescent Psychiatry, 47*(10), 1173–1181.

Peris, T. S., Sugar, C. A., Bergman, R. L., Chang, S., Langley, A., & Piacentini, J. (2012). Family factors predict treatment outcome for pediatric obsessive–compulsive disorder. *Journal of Consulting and Clinical Psychology, 80*(2), 255–263.

Piacentini, J., Peris, T., Bergman, L., Chang, S., & Jaffer, M. (2010). Functional impairment in childhood OCD: Development and psychometric properties of the Child Obsessive–Compulsive

Impact Scale—Revised (COIS-R). *Journal of Clinical Child and Adolescent Psychology, 36*(4), 645–653.

Ruscio, A. M., Stein, D. J., Chiu, W. T., & Kessler, R. C. (2010). The epidemiology of obsessive–compulsive disorder in the National Comorbidity Survey Replication. *Molecular Psychiatry, 15*(1), 53–63.

Scahill, L., Riddle, M. A., McSwiggin-Hardin, M., Ort, S. I., King, R. A., Goodman, W. K., et al. (1997). Children's Yale–Brown Obsessive Compulsive Scale: Reliability and validity. *Journal of the American Academy of Child and Adolescent Psychiatry, 36*(6), 844–852.

Schuberth, D. A., Selles, R. R., & Stewart, S. E. (2018). Coercive and disruptive behaviors mediate group cognitive-behavioral therapy response in pediatric obsessive–compulsive disorder. *Comprehensive Psychiatry, 86,* 74–81.

Selles, R. R., Belschner, L., Negreiros, J., Lin, S., Schuberth, D., McKenney, K., et al. (2018a). Group family-based cognitive behavioral therapy for pediatric obsessive compulsive disorder?: Global outcomes and predictors of improvement. *Psychiatry Research, 260,* 116–122.

Selles, R. R., Højgaard, D. R. M. A., Ivarsson, T., Thomsen, P. H., McBride, N., Storch, E. A., et al. (2018b). Symptom insight in pediatric obsessive–compulsive disorder: Outcomes of an international aggregated cross-sectional sample. *Journal of American Academy of Child and Adolescent Psychiatry, 57*(8), 615–619.

Selles, R. R., Højgaard, D. R. M. A., Ivarsson, T., Thomsen, P. H., McBride, N., Storch, E. A., et al. (2019). Avoidance, insight, impairment, recognition, concordance, and cognitive-behavioral therapy outcomes in pediatric obsessive–compulsive disorder. *Journal of the American Academy of Child and Adolescent Psychiatry.* [Epub ahead of print]

Sigra, S., Hesselmark, E., & Bejerot, S. (2018). Treatment of PANDAS and PANS: A systematic review. *Neuroscience and Biobehavioral Reviews, 86,* 51–65.

Simons, J. S., & Gaher, R. M. (2005). The Distress Tolerance Scale: Development and validation of a self-report measure. *Motivation and Emotion, 29,* 83–102.

Stewart, S. E. (2012). Rage takes center stage: Focus on an under-appreciated aspect of pediatric obsessive–compulsive disorder. *Journal of the American Academy of Child and Adolescent Psychiatry, 51*(6), 569–571.

Stewart, S. E., Beresin, C., Haddad, S., Stack, D. E., Fama, J., & Jenike, M. (2008). Predictors of family accommodation in obsessive–compulsive disorder. *Annals of Clinical Psychiatry, 20*(2), 65–70.

Stewart, S. E., Geller, D. A., Jenike, M., Pauls, D., Shaw, D., & Mullin, B. (2004). Long-term outcome of pediatric obsessive–compulsive disorder: A meta-analysis and qualitative review of the literature. *Acta Psychiatrica Scandinavica, 110*(1), 4–13.

Stewart, S. E., Hu, Y. P., Hezel, D. M., Proujansky, R., Lamstein, A., Walsh, C., et al. (2011). Development and psychometric properties of the OCD Family Functioning (OFF) Scale. *Journal of Family Psychology, 25*(3), 434–443.

Stewart, S. E., Hu, Y. P., Leung, A., Chan, E., Hezel, D. M., Lin, S. Y., et al. (2017). A multisite study of family functioning impairment in pediatric obsessive–compulsive disorder. *Journal of the American Academy of Child and Adolescent Psychiatry, 56*(3), 241–249.

Stewart, S. E., Rosario, M. C., Baer, L. E. E., Carter, A. S., Brown, T. A., Scharf, J. M., et al. (2008). Four-factor structure of obsessive–compulsive disorder symptoms in children, adolescents and adults. *Journal of the American Academy of Child and Adolescent Psychiatry, 47*(7), 763–772.

Storch, E. A., Caporino, N. E., Morgan, J. R., Lewin, A. B., Rojas, A., Brauer, L., et al. (2011). Preliminary investigation of web-camera delivered cognitive-behavioral therapy for youth with obsessive–compulsive disorder. *Psychiatry Research, 189*(3), 407–412.

Storch, E. A., Geffken, G. R., Merlo, L. J., Jacob, M. L., Murphy, T. K., Goodman, W. K., et al. (2007a). Family accommodation in pediatric obsessive–compulsive disorder. *Journal of Clinical Child and Adolescent Psychology, 36*(2), 207–216.

Storch, E. A., Geffken, G. R., Merlo, L. J., Mann, G., Duke, D., Munson, M., et al. (2007b).

Family-based cognitive-behavioral therapy for pediatric obsessive–compulsive disorder: Comparison of intensive and weekly approaches. *Journal of the American Academy of Child and Adolescent Psychiatry, 46*(4), 469–478.

Thomas, J. K., Suresh Kumar, P. N., Verma, A. N., Sinha, V. K., & Andrade, C. (2004). Psychosocial dysfunction and family burden in schizophrenia and obsessive compulsive disorder. *Indian Journal of Psychiatry, 46*(3), 238–243.

Turner, C., O'Gorman, B., Nair, A., & O'Kearney, R. (2018). Moderators and predictors of response to cognitive behaviour therapy for pediatric obsessive–compulsive disorder: A systematic review. *Psychiatry Research, 261*, 50–60.

Turrell, S. L., & Bell, M. (2016). *ACT for adolescents: Treating teens and adolescents in individual and group therapy.* Oakland, CA: Context Press.

Twohig, M. P., Abramowitz, J. S., Smith, B. M., Fabricant, L. E., Jacoby, R. J., Morrison, K. L., et al. (2018). Adding acceptance and commitment therapy to exposure and response prevention for obsessive–compulsive disorder: A randomized controlled trial. *Behaviour Research and Therapy, 108*, 1–9.

Twohig, M. P., Whittal, M. L., Cox, J. M., & Gunter, R. (2010). An initial investigation into the processes of change in ACT, CT, and ERP for OCD. *International Journal of Behavioral Consultation and Therapy, 6*(1), 67–83.

van Grootheest, D. S., Cath, D. C., Beekman, A. T., & Boomsma, D. I. (2005). Twin studies on obsessive–compulsive disorder: A review. *Twin Research and Human Genetics, 8*(5), 450–458.

Van Oppen, P., & Arntz, A. (1994). Cognitive therapy for obsessive–compulsive disorder. *Behaviour Research and Therapy, 32*(1), 79–87.

Westwell-Roper, C., & Stewart, S. E. (2019). Challenges in the diagnosis and treatment of pediatric obsessive–compulsive disorder. *Indian Journal of Psychiatry, 61*(Suppl. 1), 119–130.

Wu, M. S., Hamblin, R., Nadeau, J., Simmons, J., Smith, A., Wilson, M., et al. (2018). Quality of life and burden in caregivers of youth with obsessive–compulsive disorder presenting for intensive treatment. *Comprehensive Psychiatry, 80*, 46–56.

Index

Note. *f* or *t* following a page number indicates a figure or a table.

Academic expectations, 192, 199–201
Acceptance and commitment therapy (ACT), 27, 30–31
Accommodations, 200–201. *See also* Family accommodation
Age factors, 6, 22–24, 41–42
Aggression, 15, 146
Anxiety and anxiety disorders, 4, 9, 31–33
Arguments, 127–128, 137, 156
Assessment, 15–17
Attention-deficit/hyperactivity disorder (ADHD), 4
Avoidance
  effectiveness of ERPs and, 178–179
  establishing a reward system and, 76–77
  family accommodation and, 7, 101–102, 113–114
  how far to go in exposures and, 83
  outcomes related to, 6
  overview, 14
  setting limits for, 127, 137
Awareness, 47–48

B

Behavioral experiments, 27–28
Behavioral problems, 15, 183–184. *See also specific behaviors*
Between-session practice. *See* Homework between sessions
Blame, 49–50, 124
Booster sessions, 228
Bossing back the OCD bully technique, 100, 104–109, 112, 130–133, 168
Breaking OCD's Rules (Module 4)
  case example, 119, 123–124
  exposure games, 120–124
  the Four S's, 118–119
  handouts and worksheets for, 130–141
  homework assignments and, 128–129
  limiting family accommodation, 124–125
  reassurance seeking and, 125–128
Breathing exercises, 31, 32–33

C

Checking behavior, 4, 127, 136
Child OCD Impact Scale (COIS), 16
Children's Yale–Brown Obsessive Compulsive Scale Checklist (CY-BOC-CL), 4, 16
Children's Yale–Brown Obsessive Compulsive Scale (CY-BOCS), 16
Cleaning compulsions, 4, 127, 136. *See also* Compulsions
Clinical Global Impression Improvement Scale (CGI-I), 16
Clinical Global Impression Severity Scale (CGI-S), 16
Clomipramine, 34, 35*t*, 37
Coercive and Disruptive Behavior Scale for Pediatric OCD (CD-POC), 17
Coercive behavior, 15
Cognitive approaches, 12, 27–30, 29*f*, 30*f*
Cognitive distancing, 161
Cognitive-behavioral therapy (CBT), 7–8, 10, 24–26
Comorbidity, 4, 34
Compulsions. *See also* Rituals; Symptoms of OCD
  effectiveness of ERPs and, 178–179
  exposure games and, 120–124
  the Four S's and, 118–119
  handouts and worksheets for, 58
  increasing awareness of, 47–48
  OCD's trap and, 99–100
  overview, 3–4, 14
  psychoeducation regarding, 42–43
  punishments and, 82
  setting limits for, 127–128, 136–137
Contamination obsessions, 4, 19, 20–21. *See also* Obsessions
Coping cards, 160, 168, 172–174
Coping with doubt technique, 161–164, 166–170, 172–174. *See also* Doubt

D

Deep brain stimulation (DBS), 37
Destigmatizing OCD. *See* Stigma

Diagnosis, 3–6, 164
Dialectical behavior therapy (DBT), 10
Diaphragmatic breathing, 31, 32–33
Distraction, 182, 190
Distress ratings. *See* Fear ratings; Subjective units of distress (SUDs)
Doubt
   case example, 163–164
   dealing with, 161–164, 172–174
   effectiveness of ERPs and, 178–179
   handouts and worksheets for, 166–170

E

Empowerment activities, 197–199
Engagement, 84, 120–124
Explaining ERPs, Building an OCD Ladder, and Implementing Rewards (Module 2)
   case example, 72–75, 81
   constructing OCD Ladders, 71–72
   establishing a reward system, 75–81
   explaining ERPs to families, 70–71
   handouts and worksheets for, 86–98
   homework assignments and, 84–85
   how far to go in exposures, 82–84
   punishments and, 82
Exposure and response prevention (ERP). *See also* Treatment
   alternatives to or delaying, 10–11
   based on age group, 22–24
   based on symptom type, 19–22
   based on treatment setting, 24–26
   complementary approaches to, 27–37
   establishing a reward system and, 75–76
   exposure games, 120–124
   handouts and worksheets for, 166–176
   how far to go in exposures, 82–84
   during the maintenance phase of treatment, 228
   overview, 7–10, 11–12, 39
   preparing for, 13–18, 48–49, 52
   psychoeducation regarding, 44–45, 92
   strategies to help with, 161–165
   troubleshooting, 177–185
Exposures, 19–22, 82–84, 162–163. *See also* Exposure and response prevention (ERP); Imaginal exposure; *In vivo* exposure
Externalizing OCD, 43–44, 49–50

F

Family. *See also* Family accommodation; Parental involvement in treatment
   coaching parents on what to do and what not to do, 51–52
   ERPs with young children and, 23
   establishing a reward system and, 75–81
   externalizing OCD, 43–44, 49–50
   handouts and worksheets for, 64–67, 92–98, 111–117
   impact of OCD on, 7
   medication and, 35
   self-care and, 53
   treatment and, 7–8
Family accommodation. *See also* Family
   case example, 102–103
   effectiveness of ERPs and, 179
   handouts and worksheets for, 111–116, 135–139, 189–194
   identifying, 100–103
   limiting, 124–125, 127–128
   overview, 7, 14, 113–114, 135–136
   treatment refusers and, 184–185
   types of, 101–102
Family Accommodation Scale (FAS), 16–17
Family-based group approach, 25. *See also* Group-based treatment
Fear ratings, 9, 24, 45–47
Fear response, 9, 83, 178–179
Feelings Thermometer, 46. *See also* OCD Ruler; Subjective units of distress (SUDs)
Floating on by strategy, 161, 168, 172–174
Foundational Treatment Tools (Module 3)
   bossing back the OCD bully technique, 100
   case example, 102–103
   family accommodation and reassurance seeking, 100–103
   handouts and worksheets for, 104–117
   homework assignments and, 103
   overview, 99
   psychoeducation regarding OCD and, 99–100
Four S's
   case example, 119
   handouts and worksheets for, 130–133, 135
   limiting family accommodation and, 124
   overview, 118–119, 135
Future planning, 211–216, 217–226

G

Games, 24, 25, 120–124
Graduation (Module 10)
   handouts and worksheets for, 230–241
   overview, 227–229
   preparing for, 213–215, 214*f*, 215*f*, 216*f*, 223–224
Group-based treatment, 24–25

H

Habituation, 8, 9
Handouts and worksheets
   Explaining ERPs, Building an OCD Ladder, and Implementing Rewards (Module 2), 86–98
   Preparing for the Future (Module 9), 217–226
   Self- and Family Care (Module 8), 202–210
   Tools to Help with ERPs (Module 6), 166–176
   Tools to Help with OCD "Bad Thoughts" (Module 5), 148–159
   Treatment Preparation (Module 1), 55–69
   Troubleshooting ERPs (Module 7), 186–194
Homework between sessions
   Breaking OCD's Rules (Module 4), 128–129, 134
   case example, 81
   compliance with, 76–77
   establishing a reward system and, 75–81
   Explaining ERPs, Building an OCD Ladder, and Implementing Rewards (Module 2), 84–85, 96
   Foundational Treatment Tools (Module 3), 103, 109–110, 116
   overview, 39
   Preparing for the Future (Module 9), 217
   Self- and Family Care (Module 8), 202
   therapist pitfalls and, 181–182
   Tools to Help with ERPs (Module 6), 165, 171
   Tools to Help with OCD "Bad Thoughts" (Module 5), 147, 152–153
   Treatment Preparation (Module 1), 53–54
   Troubleshooting ERPs (Module 7), 185, 188

Index

I

Imaginal exposure
  case example, 144–145
  dealing with doubts and, 162–163
  handouts and worksheets for, 148–151, 154–157
  overview, 142–146, 154
  when to use, 20
In vivo exposure
  dealing with doubts and, 162–163
  examples of, 20–22
  imaginal exposures and, 145–146
  when to use, 19–20
Individualized education plan (IEP), 200–201
Inflated responsibility, 28–29, 29*f*
Intrusive thoughts. *See also* Obsessions; Symptoms of OCD
  dealing with doubts and, 162–163
  handouts and worksheets for, 154–157
  imaginal exposures and, 142–146
  overestimation of threats and, 29–30, 30*f*
  overview, 4

L

Limit setting, 124–128, 135–139

M

Maintenance, 228. *See also* Relapse prevention
Medication, 10, 27, 33–37, 35*t*, 37, 224
Modules, treatment, 11–12, 39. *See also individual modules*
Motivation, 75–81, 120–124, 197–198

N

Negative interactions, 127–128, 137, 156
Negative reinforcement, 99–100
Normal behaviors, 27–28
"Not-right" feelings, 20, 122

O

Obsessions. *See also* Intrusive thoughts; Symptoms of OCD
  dealing with doubts and, 162–163
  examples of *in vivo* exposures, 20–22
  handouts and worksheets for, 58
  imaginal exposures and, 142–146
  increasing awareness of, 47–48
  OCD's trap and, 99–100
  overview, 3–4
  psychoeducation regarding, 42–43
  reassurance seeking and, 125–128
Obsessive–compulsive disorder (OCD) in general, 3–7
Obsessive–compulsive-related disorders (OCRDs), 5
OCD bully's trap, 99–100, 104–108, 111–112, 130–133, 166–170, 241. *See also* Bossing back the OCD bully technique
OCD Family Function Scale Part 1 (OFF), 17
OCD Ladder
  case example, 72–75
  construction of, 71–72, 73–74
  handouts and worksheets for, 86–89, 92, 239
  moving up too fast or too slow, 180–181
OCD Ruler. *See also* Subjective units of distress (SUDs)
  construction of the OCD Ladder and, 73–74
  handouts and worksheets for, 61–62, 66
  overview, 45–47
OCD-related rage. *See* Rage
Outcomes, 6, 15–18, 45
Overestimation of threat, 29–30, 30*f*

P

PANDAS. *See* Pediatric autoimmune neuropsychiatric disorders associated with streptococcal infections (PANDAS)
PANS. *See* Pediatric acute-onset neuropsychiatric syndrome (PANS)
Parent Tolerance of Their Child's Distress (PT-CD), 17
Parental accommodations. *See* Family accommodation
Parental involvement in treatment. *See also* Family
  clarifying parent's role, 50–53
  ERPs with young children and, 23–24
  establishing a reward system and, 75–81
  externalizing OCD and limiting blame and, 49–50
  group treatment and, 25
  handouts and worksheets for, 64–67, 68–69, 92–98, 111–117, 135–141, 154–159, 172–176, 189–194, 206–210, 223–226, 234–236
  medication and, 35
  OCD-related rage and, 146
  overview, 39
  preparing for ERPs, 48–49, 52
  self-care and, 53
Pediatric acute-onset neuropsychiatric syndrome (PANS), 5–6, 37
Pediatric autoimmune neuropsychiatric disorders associated with streptococcal infections (PANDAS), 5, 37
Pediatric obsessive–compulsive disorder (OCD) in general, 3–7
Perfectionism, 195–197, 206
Practice between sessions. *See* Homework between sessions
Preparing for the Future (Module 9)
  consolidating gains, 212–213
  handouts and worksheets for, 217–226
  homework assignments and, 216
  overview, 211
  preparations for the end of treatment, 213–215, 214*f*, 215*f*, 216*f*
  warning signs and anticipating symptom exacerbations, 211–212
Pretreatment assessments and checklists, 15–18
Progressive muscle relaxation (PMR), 31
Psychoeducation
  differentiating between obsessions and compulsions, 41, 42–43
  explaining ERPs to families, 70–71
  explaining OCD, 41–42
  externalizing OCD, 41, 43–44
  handouts and worksheets for, 55–67
  OCD's trap, 99–100
  regarding treatment, 41
Punishments, 82

R

Rage, 15, 146, 154–157
Ratings of fear. *See* Fear ratings; Subjective units of distress (SUDs)
Readiness for ERPs, 15–18
Reassurance giving, 7, 101–102, 113–114, 179–180. *See also* Family accommodation
Reassurance seeking
  dealing with doubts and, 162
  identifying, 100–103
  overview, 125–128
  school setting and, 200
  therapist pitfalls, 179–180
Refusals
  homework assignments and, 76–77
  how far to go in exposures and, 83–84

Refusals (cont.)
  overview, 184–185
  therapist pitfalls and, 181–182
  as a treatment-interfering behavior, 184
Relapse prevention
  handouts and worksheets for, 217–226
  overview, 211–216, 223
  parents' role in, 224
Relaxation training, 31–33
Reluctance to engage in exposures, 83–84. *See also* Refusals
Repetitive transcranial magnetic stimulation (rTMS), 36
Residential treatment, 26
Responsibilities, daily, 101, 113, 191
Responsibility, inflated, 28–29, 29f
Reward systems
  case example, 81
  ERPs with young children and, 23
  establishing, 75–81
  handouts and worksheets for, 92–95
  therapist pitfalls and, 181
Risk taking, 186–187
Rituals. *See also* Compulsions
  effectiveness of ERPs and, 178–179
  exposure games and, 120–124
  family accommodation and, 101–102, 113–114
  the Four S's and, 118–119
  limiting family accommodation, 124–125
  OCD's trap and, 99–100
  overview, 14
  psychoeducation regarding, 42–43
  punishments and, 82
  relaxation training and, 31–32
  setting limits for, 127–128, 136–137
Routines, 102, 114

S

Safety behaviors, 28, 179, 191
School setting, 199–201
Self- and Family Care (Module 8)
  boosting self-esteem, 195–197
  empowerment activities, 197–199
  handouts and worksheets for, 202–210
  homework assignments and, 201
  overview, 195
  school setting, 199–201
  self-care for parents, 199
Self-care for parents, 53, 195, 199, 207
Self-esteem, 195–197, 202–204, 206
Somatic approaches to treatment, 27, 33–37, 35t

SSRIs. *See also* Medication
  overview, 10, 34–35, 35t
  PANDAS and PANS and, 37
  side effects of, 36
Stigma, 35–36, 164, 172–174
Subjective units of distress (SUDs), 9, 24, 45–47
Symptoms of OCD. *See also* Compulsions; Intrusive thoughts; Obsessions; *individual symptoms*
  fine-tuning ERP based on, 19–22
  monitoring, 47–48
  outcomes related to, 6
  overview, 3–4
  PANDAS and PANS and, 5–6
  warning signs of symptom return, 211–212

T

Technology-based CBT, 24
Therapist pitfalls, 179–183
Thoughts, intrusive. *See* Intrusive thoughts
Threat, overestimation of, 29–30, 30f
Tics and tic disorders, 4, 10
Tools to Help with ERPs (Module 6)
  case example, 163–164
  coping cards, 160
  dealing with doubts, 161–164
  floating on by strategy, 161
  handouts and worksheets for, 166–176
  homework assignments and, 165
  OCD disclosure and reducing stigma, 164
Tools to Help with OCD "Bad Thoughts" (Module 5)
  handouts and worksheets for, 148–159
  homework assignments and, 147
  imaginal exposures, 142–146
  OCD-related rage, 146
Treatment. *See also* Exposure and response prevention (ERP); *individual modules*
  behaviors that interfere with, 183–184
  obstacles to, 14–15
  overview, 7–8, 11–12, 39
  PANDAS and PANS and, 37
  preparing parents for, 48–49
  pretreatment assessments and checklists and, 15–18
  primarily cognitive approaches, 27–30, 29f, 30f
  psychoeducation regarding, 41
  setting characteristics, 24–26

  therapist pitfalls, 179–183
  treatment planning, 13–14
Treatment Preparation (Module 1)
  clarifying parent's role, 50–53
  externalizing OCD and limiting blame, 49–50
  handouts and worksheets for, 55–59
  homework assignments, 53–54
  monitoring symptoms, 47–48
  preparing parents for treatment, 48–53
  psychoeducation component, 41–45
  using the OCD Ruler and, 45–47
Treatment-interfering behaviors (TIBs), 183–184
Tricyclic antidepressant (TCA), 34, 35t, 37. *See also* Medication
Triggers
  behavioral problems and, 15
  exposure and response prevention (ERP) and, 7–8, 179
  family accommodation and, 7
  neutralizing of core fears and, 14
  overview, 14
  relaxation training and, 31–32
  school setting and, 200
Troubleshooting ERPs (Module 7)
  effectiveness of ERPs, 178–179
  handouts and worksheets for, 186–194
  homework assignments and, 185
  overview, 177
  therapist pitfalls, 179–183
  treatment refusers, 184–185
  treatment-interfering behaviors, 183–184

U

Uncertainty
  case example, 163–164
  dealing with, 161–164
  effectiveness of ERPs and, 178–179
  exposure games and, 121–122
  fine-tuning ERP based on, 20
  handouts and worksheets for, 166–170
  therapist pitfalls, 180

W

Warning signs, 211–212
Washing rituals, 127, 136
Worksheets. *See* Handouts and worksheets
Worry scripts, 142–144, 148–151, 153, 154–157